Alternatives to Antibiotics

Alternatives to Antibiotics

Dr John McKenna

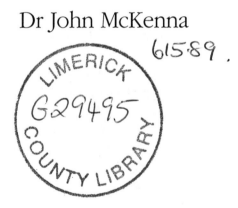
GILL & MACMILLAN

Gill & Macmillan Ltd
Goldenbridge
Dublin 8
with associated companies throughout the world
© John McKenna 1996
0 7171 2469 X

Index compiled by Helen Litton

Print origination by O'K Graphic Design, Dublin

Printed by ColourBooks Ltd, Dublin

A catalogue record for this book is available from
the British Library.

1 3 5 4 2

This book is dedicated to four very special people in my life—
Charity, Jackie, Marianne and David—my children.

Contents

Foreword

It was after a talk in Dublin that I first had the pleasure of meeting Dr John McKenna. During our conversation, John told me he was writing this book—its publication could not have come at a more important time. It is a long-awaited and necessary book which addresses many issues and answers many questions.

Nowadays, people have a better understanding of the side effects related to the long-term use of antibiotics. Back in 1958, when I graduated in pharmacy, it was not an issue of public concern. The issue was in my mind even then, however. At that particular time there was an explosion in the use of antibiotics, tranquillisers and sleeping tablets. Since then, development of these drugs has continued unabated and today, when I look at the numerous patients I treat in my seven British clinics, I understand even better what I saw happening in the late fifties.

This book describes the many alternatives available. Echinacea, for example, was recently shown to be one of the best natural antibiotics in a study at the University of München in Germany. My own partner, Dr Alfred Vogel, now ninety-five years old and still skiing, has been promoting Echinacea for more than forty years and I am delighted that he can now see a scientific report validating the great benefits of Echinacea. This report proves that there *are* natural ways to support and boost the defences of the human body.

Some time ago I was asked to speak to a group of doctors and medical students in Germany. While talking about the immune system, I briefly mentioned a product called Echinaforce, the fresh herb extract from *Echinacea purpurea*. The doctors in question were very interested in the methods I have been using, during the past thirty-five years, to help human suffering. I was especially pleased when at the end of my lecture one doctor stood up to endorse what I had said about Echinacea. Apparently, while travelling in Brazil she had acquired a nasty throat infection. As there was no pharmacy nearby she was unable to obtain antibiotics, so she bought a bottle of Echinaforce in a simple health food store instead. She took twice the recommended dosage as she believed it could not do the job and found, to her surprise, that her sore throat had eased considerably by evening. Since then she has prescribed Echinacea to many of her patients, with great success.

This clear and concisely written book is a timely reminder of the great possibilities that nature has to offer. Nature is balanced and will always have the power to heal. The many subjects that Dr John McKenna has discussed in this book open the way to a greater recognition and understanding of natural remedies. After all, we are born in nature and have to obey the laws of nature if we want to stay healthy and fit. I am happy to see more and more people throughout the world becoming aware of the natural options available to them, instead of using and abusing synthetic antibiotics.

I am sure that the readers of this book will be impressed and rewarded by the tremendous research and knowledge that has gone in to its publication.

Jan de Vries D.Ho.Med.,
D.O.M.R.O., N.D.M.R.N., D.Ac., M.B.Ac.A.

Preface

Here are the clinical records of a fourteen-year-old boy. He was born in January 1980. Each asterisk (*) highlights the use of an antibiotic.

Date	Prescription	Type of drug
09/1980*	Keflex	Antibiotic
01/1981*	Septrin	Antibiotic
05/1981	Piriton	Anti-histamine
07/1981*	Pen-V	Antibiotic
12/1981*	Bactrim	Antibiotic
01/1982*	Bactrim	Antibiotic
03/1982*	Keflex	Antibiotic
05/1982*	Amoxil	Antibiotic
09/1982*	Penbritin	Antibiotic
04/1983*	Keflex	Antibiotic
04/1983*	Amoxil	Antibiotic
06/1983*	Erythroped	Antibiotic
08/1983*	Amoxil	Antibiotic
08/1983	Hydrocortisone cream	Steroid
09/1983*	Erythroped	Antibiotic
	Maxolon	Anti-nausea drug
10/1983*	Keflex	Antibiotic
11/1983	Hydrocortisone cream	Steroid
12/1983	Vallergan syrup	Anti-histamine
01/1984*	Keflex	Antibiotic
04/1984*	Keflex	Antibiotic
06/1984*	Keflex	Antibiotic
	Alupent	Bronchodilator
	(to dilate the airways in asthmatics)	
07/1984*	Keflex	Antibiotic
09/1984*	Erythroped	Antibiotic
10/1984	Diprosone cream	Potent steroid

11/1984	Vallergan	Anti-histamine
12/1984*	Ceporex	Antibiotic
01/1985*	Ceporex	Antibiotic
	Diprosone cream	Potent steroid
02/1985*	Amoxil	Antibiotic
06/1985*	Amoxil	Antibiotic
07/1985	Triludan syrup	Anti-histamine
09/1985*	Keflex	Antibiotic
	Ventolin	Bronchodilator
10/1985*	Distaclor	Antibiotic
	Ventolin	Bronchodilator
11/1985*	Amoxil	Antibiotic
	Ventolin	Bronchodilator
12/1985*	Amoxil	Antibiotic
01/1986	Hydrocortisone cream	Steroid
01/1986*	Fucidin cream	Antibiotic
01/1986*	Ceporex	Antibiotic
02/1986*	Keflex	Antibiotic
	Ventolin	Bronchodilator
03/1986	Ventolin	Bronchodilator
03/1986	Ventolin	Bronchodilator
04/1986	Ventolin	Bronchodilator
04/1986*	Erythroped	Antibiotic

This child was given his first antibiotic when he was nine months old. Before he had reached his seventh birthday, he had received no less than *thirty* courses of antibiotics. He was diagnosed as being asthmatic in September 1985.

These antibiotics were prescribed for sore throats, coughs, bronchitis, and as a 'precaution' when the child had a wheezy chest. The steroids were prescribed for allergic rashes—which may well have been caused by the antibiotics!

This senseless use of antibiotics—one course after the next, after the next, after the next—must be condemned. Remember, this is a young child who was being given these drugs. It could have been *your* child and, as this book will show you, these drugs are far from harmless.

This, however, is not the worst case I have encountered. I

am alarmed by this. As a patient, parent or interested reader, you are probably alarmed too. *You* are the ones who have alerted me to this problem and who have asked me for a better method of treatment.

Early in 1994, I gave a series of talks entitled 'How to treat infections without antibiotics'. These talks attracted considerable attention, so much so that it became apparent to me that people wanted to know a lot more about this subject. It was at these talks that I was encouraged to put my approach on paper—hence this book.

I do not quote the above case history to criticise the medical profession, the child's doctor or his parents. Nor do I seek to lay blame at anyone's feet or to frighten you. Rather, I want to highlight the inherent difficulty in trying to treat infections with antibiotics alone. Believe me, there are safe, effective alternatives available. Don't take my word for this. Instead, open your mind and read the research. Above all, try the alternatives. It is only by trying alternatives that you will learn for yourself, as I have had to. I am privileged to have had such wonderful patients who have continuously supported me in my work through their understanding, their belief and their patience. They have taught me much, especially about myself, and I thank them.

This boy's case history suggests that a more broad-minded approach to the causes of recurrent infections is needed. Treating the symptoms is often fruitless, and does damage to everyone concerned. Locating the underlying causes is the only way to treat such a child. This child's case also reflects the need for a less scientific, and a more human, caring and compassionate approach to medicine. Put another way—more of the heart and less of the head! The head without the heart results in a form of medicine which is cold and unsympathetic to human suffering. It lacks wisdom and understanding as to the consequences of treating people in this way. The global problem of resistance to antibiotics would not have arisen if we had placed more emphasis on this wisdom and understanding, and less on accepted scientific knowledge. Knowledge, when guided by the wisdom handed down to us from past generations, will guarantee a future. But to accept and understand this wisdom, you must open your heart.

Many doctors know very little about alternative medicine, yet they are quick to say that it does not work. For example, while at the Royal Victoria Hospital in Belfast, I heard a consultant surgeon from Scotland condemn acupuncture as nonsense and quackery. This is sad to hear! The research done to date clearly shows that acupuncture does work.

It is important that you and I speak from the heart and say what we feel is right, even in the face of aggressive contradiction. It is also important to convert your local doctor and continually insist on safer medicine. The same message, heard repeatedly and from different sources, eventually has an impact. If you say nothing, medicine will not change. Then you, or your child, may be the recipient of the kind of treatment described earlier. It is time for you to choose.

A safer form of medicine and a gentler approach to patients are what I stand for. If this is what you stand for, then say so. By doing this, you encourage change to occur. I believe in people: the more information and power people have, the more common sense will prevail. The purpose of this book is to inform people about the medical issues confronting us today. I hope you will both enjoy it and learn more by reading it.

Dr John McKenna

Acknowledgments

I would like to thank my good friend, David Niket Ring, for helping to guide me through a very difficult period in my life. His wisdom has enabled me to see the importance of making certain changes, including writing this book and expressing what I feel more publicly.

I would also like to thank another friend, Angela Leahy, for her constant encouragement and belief in me and for helping me with many aspects of the preparation of the original draft.

My practice nurse, Joan Deegan, also deserves thanks for helping me to keep the practice going while I was working such long hours on this book. Her care, compassion, understanding and common sense made it a pleasure to work with her.

Thanks also go to Siobhán for her pleasant approach, for covering for Joan and for making it possible for me to get on with my research. My thanks to John Doyle for many things, especially for proof-reading the final script.

I did not realise the importance of a good editor until I worked with both Roberta Reeners and Karin Whooley. In spite of having little medical knowledge, they helped me to get my message across in a simple and effective way. My apologies to Aisling Collins for not being able to use her evocative illustrations this time.

Thanks to Wendy MacDonnell and to Hansen Laboratories for their help with research information; to Merck, Sharp and Dohme for the use of *Antibiotics in Historical Perspective*; and to Schaper and Brümmer for help with research and for slides of certain herbs.

I am grateful to all my patients for their support over the past five years. It is because of them that this book came about. Without their help, a simpler and gentler form of medicine would not be possible. Particular thanks to those who agreed to let me use their case histories.

My greatest debt of gratitude is to my family, who have borne the pain of long periods of separation with great strength.

Introduction

Antibiotics are drugs which are used to treat infections. Initially developed in the 1940s, a whole range of antibiotics have been produced since then and they are now among the most commonly prescribed drugs in the world.

Antibiotics act by killing, or controlling the growth of, the germ which is causing the disease. They are very effective in combating infections caused by bacteria—like a streptococcal sore throat, for example. They are absolutely *useless* in treating infections caused by viruses, such as influenza or the common cold.

The real value of antibiotics is in sharp decline today because of the massive worldwide abuse of these substances. Reports in recent years show an ever-increasing problem of resistance to antibiotics emerging in different parts of the world. As people become more aware of this and of the side-effects of antibiotics, they are demanding alternatives. This book describes those alternatives in detail. Natural medicines, especially herbal and homeopathic medicines, are coming back in vogue and are regaining their rightful place in providing a balanced way of treating infection. People are becoming much more conscious of the foods they eat and are aware of the need for food supplements, especially vitamins and minerals. All of these topics, as well as case histories to illustrate the way in which specific infections can be treated by natural means, make this book a valuable asset for any household. It is especially important for the parents of children who suffer from recurrent infections.

Since this book is aimed at the general public, it has been kept as simple as possible, with the minimum of scientific or medical jargon. It is designed to show that it is possible to treat infections without antibiotics, but it also emphasises the fact that antibiotics may sometimes be needed. This, however, is the exception rather than the rule. The book is not suggesting that you stay away from your doctor. Rather, you should visit him/her and encourage him/her to use natural methods whenever possible.

When choosing a doctor, try to find one who has been trained in using natural methods as well as conventional medicine. Since many of the medicines discussed in this book will only be available on prescription (according to European legislation implemented in 1995), it is best to go to practitioners who can prescribe them.

The aim of this book is to bring some common sense back into clinical medicine and to support a gentler way of healing people. The first part of the book deals with the history and development of antibiotics, their conventional usage, and the much-publicised issue of antibiotic resistance. Later, I deal with some of the common infections in children. The greater part of the book, however, looks at alternative methods of treating infections, from herbal medicine to homeopathy to nutritional medicine.

The case histories have been selected from my own practice for the purpose of illustrating my particular point of view. (All the names have been changed to protect the confidentiality of the patients concerned.) I could include many cases of a more dramatic nature, such as the one at the beginning of the book. However, I have chosen to keep the case histories simple so that they do not overshadow my purpose in writing—to illustrate the value of the different forms of alternative medicine in treating infections.

1

The History of Antibiotics

'The gold rush'

From early times to the nineteenth century

The earliest evidence of humans using plants, or other natural substances, for therapeutic use comes from the Neanderthal period over 50,000 years ago. In northern Iraq, archaeologists uncovered evidence of human remains which had been buried with a range of herbs, some of which are now known to be antibacterial.[1] Many of these herbs are still used by the inhabitants of this region today.

HONEY

The first prescription for treating infections may well have come from the Egyptians around 1550 BC. Written as *mrht*, *byt* and *ftt*, it was a mixture of lard, honey and lint and was used as an ointment for dressing wounds.

We know that honey is antibacterial—it kills bacterial cells by drawing water out of them. In addition, the enzyme inhibine, which is found in honey, converts glucose and oxygen into hydrogen peroxide, a well-known disinfectant.

At the present time, I have a patient who has surface wounds on the ankles, wrists and elbows. These wounds are very resistant to treatment with antibiotics, but honey heals them with little difficulty. I have found that honey is also excellent for treating infected varicose ulcers.

[1] An antibacterial is any substance used to kill bacteria or to prevent them from multiplying.

1

Tincta in melle linamenta was a regular prescription in Roman times. It is essentially the same ointment as the Egyptians used, with honey as the active ingredient. The Greeks also used honey in wound dressings, often combining it with copper oxide.

More recently, during World War II, an ointment of honey and lard was used in Shanghai to treat wounds and skin infections, and with very good results.

GARLIC AND ONIONS

Honey was not the only antibacterial substance used by the Egyptians. Fragrant resins, such as frankincense and myrrh, were used to preserve human remains. Onions have often been found in the body cavities of mummies, as they are also antibacterial.

The anti-infective properties of onions and garlic were confirmed by researchers in the 1940s. A substance called allicin was isolated and this was shown to be highly effective in killing bacteria.

Another plant, the radish, is also thought to have been used therapeutically by the Egyptians. The anti-infective property of this plant was confirmed with the isolation of raphanin, a substance which has significant antibacterial activity against a broad range of infections.

MOULDS

The work of Alexander Fleming in the 1920s showed that moulds, such as *Penicillium spp.*, can produce antibacterial chemicals. But the use of moulds dates back to the Egyptians, and perhaps even earlier. An Egyptian physician, quoted in the Ebers Papyrus around 1550 BC, stated that if a 'wound rots . . . then bind on it spoiled barley bread'. Indeed, the Egyptians used all kinds of moulds to treat surface infections. The ancient Chinese also used moulds to treat boils, carbuncles and other skin infections.

WINE AND VINEGAR

Wine and vinegar have been popular treatments for infected wounds since the time of Hippocrates. Vinegar is an acid and a powerful antiseptic (a chemical which kills all germs, including viruses and bacteria). The antibacterial properties of wine cannot be fully attributed to its alcohol content, as this is very low. Recent chemical analysis of wine, however, has brought to light the presence of an antibacterial substance called malvoside and it is this substance which is now thought to give wine its antibacterial properties.

COPPER

Inorganic substances have also been used to treat infections throughout the ages. Copper was widely used by the Egyptians, Greeks and Romans, often in combination with honey. Modern scientific tests have proven that copper is indeed antibacterial. For example, a skin infection known as impetigo which is caused by *Staphylococcus aureus*, is currently being treated in France with *Eau Dalibour*, a combination of zinc and copper. This prescription dates from the time of Jacques Dalibour, surgeon general of the army of Louis XIV, but it may well have been part of French folk medicine long before this.

ANTIBIOTICS IN ANCIENT AFRICA

In his book, *The Antibiotic Paradox*, Dr Stuart Levy mentions the recent discovery in Africa of 1000-year-old mummies on which traces of tetracycline (a modern antibiotic) were found. Some of the grains used by these people also contained traces of tetracycline and micro-organisms producing this antibiotic were found in soil samples taken from the area. Had these people discovered tetracycline and used it over the centuries? If so, why was bacterial resistance not a problem for them— or was it?

The nineteenth and early twentieth centuries

GOOD BACTERIA

During the nineteenth century, various experiments were done in an attempt to find a magic, powerful antibacterial substance that would rid humankind of the scourge of infection. In 1877, experiments in Paris demonstrated the benefits of using harmless, 'good' bacteria to treat pathogenic

3

or harmful bacteria. These experiments did indeed prove that harmless bacteria could be used to compete with pathogens (harmful bacteria), although they did not kill the pathogens.

Also in Paris, Louis Pasteur described the beneficial effects of injecting animals with harmless soil bacteria to combat anthrax. Many other experiments on anthrax and cholera confirmed these findings and proved that harmless bacteria can inhibit the growth of disease-causing bacteria. Later in this book, you will read about the beneficial effects of 'live' yoghurt which contains 'good' bacteria. These 'good' bacteria assist the body by producing certain vitamins while at the same time protecting the body against the growth of harmful, disease-causing bacteria.

PYOCYANASE

In Germany in 1888, an antibacterial substance called pyocyanase was isolated. Animal trials of this substance showed it to be very effective. In fact, the results were so exciting that trials were undertaken in humans suffering from a variety of infections. However, the results of the human trials were very disappointing—pyocyanase was found to be too toxic. Consequently, all research on this substance halted.

SALVARSAN

In 1910, a more promising agent called salvarsan (a dye) was shown to be effective in the treatment of syphilis, a common sexually-transmitted disease at the time. Again, toxicity in humans was a major barrier to its development and widespread use.

The problem of toxicity and the failure to find other anti-microbial agents were the two factors hindering the progress of researchers. Enthusiasm began to wane in the search for the 'magic bullet' that would rid humanity of infectious diseases, many of which were major causes of death at this time.

THE PENICILLIN ERA

All of this changed, however, in 1928 when Alexander

Fleming discovered penicillin. After distinguishing himself in his medical studies, Dr Fleming started research work in pathology in 1908. His early work led to the isolation of lysozyme, an enzyme in human tears and nasal mucus. This enzyme proved to be mildly antibacterial, but it was not very effective against most human infections.

In 1928, while attempting to grow *Staphylococcus spp.* on an agar plate, Fleming noticed that the growth of this bacterium was inhibited by a mould which had accidentally contaminated the plate. He decided to identify the mould, which was eventually called *Penicillium notatum*. Fleming was excited by this discovery. He cultured the mould in a special broth and injected the broth into some of his patients who had various infectious diseases. The results were encouraging and the broth proved to be non-toxic. Unfortunately though, Fleming had not made enough of this broth and when he presented a paper on his findings in 1929, his colleagues in the medical profession were not particularly impressed or interested.

It took two other gifted researchers, Drs Florey and Chain, working in Oxford University in the late 1930s and early 1940s, to realise the importance of Dr Fleming's findings. It was their pioneering work that brought penicillin into clinical use.

Florey, an Australian doctor, had come to Oxford on a scholarship to study pathology. Chain was a German chemist who had fled from the Nazis in the 1930s and had ended up in England.

Florey was eager to form a group of researchers who were interested in finding effective antibacterial substances. He was the microbiologist and clinician, while Chain was the chemist capable of isolating, purifying and studying the properties of potential antibacterial substances. Their research team was made up of twenty of the best scientists in Britain at the time. They focused their attention on the work of Alexander Fleming and worked at purifying penicillin and testing its effectiveness.

In one laboratory experiment, the team injected fifty mice with a lethal dose of *Streptococci spp.* Twenty-five of these animals received frequent injections of penicillin. The control group (the other twenty-five mice) was not injected with penicillin. After ten days, twenty-four of the twenty-five penicillin-treated mice had survived. All mice in the control group were dead. These startling results were reported in the well-known medical journal, *The Lancet*, on 24 August 1940.

In 1941, the Oxford group conducted their first clinical trial of penicillin. Their patient was a 43-year-old policeman who was suffering from septicaemia (blood poisoning). The man was dying, so Florey and Chain decided to inject penicillin intra-muscularly every three hours, for five days. Within twenty-four hours, there was a marked improvement in the man's condition. By the fourth day, his fever was gone and he was eating again. However, after the fifth day, the supply of penicillin ran out and the patient's condition started to deteriorate again. He eventually died. Despite his death, it was clear to all that penicillin was extremely effective at fighting infection.

The Oxford group's next challenge was finding a way to produce penicillin in large, economical quantities. All efforts to get industrial support for their research in Britain were fruitless and in the summer of 1941, they went to the U.S. Here they succeeded in getting a number of pharmaceutical companies involved in the industrial production of penicillin, including Merck, Squibb, Pfizer, Abbott, Winthrop and Commercial Solvents. It was these American pharmaceutical companies that made penicillin a therapeutic reality.

Subsequent clinical trials produced spectacular results. Penicillin demonstrated remarkable effectiveness against a range of infections, including pneumonia, septicaemia, scarlet fever, 'strep' throat, diphtheria, gonorrhoea and rheumatic fever. There was a general belief that it could help treat any disease—a myth which still exists today! Tremendous publicity surrounded this new 'miracle drug' and in 1945, Fleming, Florey and Chain were jointly awarded the Nobel Prize in Physiology and Medicine.

Penicillin was later produced in oral form and was added to many products, including salves, throat lozenges, nasal ointments, and cosmetic creams. Prior to 1955, its sale was not controlled so anyone could buy it over the counter without a prescription. This excessive and uncontrolled use led to the overgrowth of resistant bacteria in the bowel (*E. coli* and *Candida spp.*). By 1955, most nations began to restrict the sale of penicillin but the damage had already been done. Resistance had become a major problem and epidemics of staphylococcal-resistant infections began to emerge in hospitals.

STREPTOMYCIN

Microbiologists have long known that soil contains very few bacteria which are capable of causing infections in humans. The study of soil bacteria, and the reasons why they are not more pathogenic to man, was the lifelong work of Selman Waksman, a research scientist at Rutgers University in New Jersey.

In 1939, Merck and Company provided Waksman with financial assistance to mount a search for antibiotics in soil micro-organisms. In 1943, this search culminated in the isolation of streptomycin, the first antibiotic to offer hope to patients with tuberculosis (TB). This antibiotic is still used today in the treatment of TB. After clinical use in TB patients, it was soon realised that streptomycin caused side-effects not seen with penicillin, including kidney damage and deafness.

However, the main problem encountered in the use of streptomycin, and the one which restricted its effectiveness, was resistance. The speed at which bacteria were able to develop resistance to the drug was a surprise to Waksman and his co-workers. Because of this, they were prompted to search for other antibiotics. This search resulted in the development of neomycin, a drug commonly used in antibacterial ointments today.

CHLORAMPHENICOL

In late 1947, the antibiotic chloramphenicol was used in a clinical trial to treat an epidemic of typhus in Bolivia. Its success in curbing the epidemic led to its use on the other side of the world—treating scrub typhus in Malaysia.

In the Bolivian epidemic, all twenty-two patients who

received chloramphenicol recovered. Of the fifty patients for whom the antibiotic was unavailable, fourteen died. The trial in Bolivia is not the only South American link with this antibiotic. Chloramphenicol was first isolated from a soil sample in Caracas, Venezuela, a discovery which was important in two ways. Firstly, it identified a new antibiotic substance and secondly, as the clinical trial showed, it could cure previously untreatable diseases, such as typhus. Later, this same antibiotic showed remarkable results in the treatment of typhoid fever. At last scientists were finding effective substances which could treat serious infections.

The euphoria which surrounded the discovery of chloramphenicol was dampened somewhat when it was shown to cause serious side-effects. By 1950, many investigators had become alarmed by the mounting evidence linking it with serious blood disorders, including anaemias and leukaemias.

Today, the use of chloramphenicol is limited in developed countries where more expensive but safer drugs are available. In developing countries, however, it is still widely used because it is so cheap to produce. It is used mainly for typhus, typhoid fever, meningitis and brucellosis, but it can also be used for other infections. You may have used it yourself—as ear drops or eye drops.

THE CEPHALOSPORINS

In the mid-1940s Giuseppe Brotzu, rector of the University of Cagliari in Sardinia, isolated an antibiotic-like substance from a mould. He conducted clinical trials with the substance (albeit in an impure form) and achieved very good results, particularly in the treatment of staphylococcal infections and in typhoid fever.

Brotzu published his results in 1948 and his work came to the attention of Florey's research group in Oxford. When they obtained samples of the fungus, they were able to isolate and purify several penicillin-like antibiotics. These were called cephalosporins. The cephalosporins are very effective in treating a wide range of bacterial infections. They destroy bacteria in a manner similar to penicillin and are valuable alternatives, especially where resistance to penicillin is a problem. The added advantage is that they have very low toxicity, although allergic reactions develop in about 5% of patients.

Modifications of the basic cephalosporin chemical structure led to the development of a whole range of these antibiotics for clinical use. Research into the development of new cephalosporins continues today.

THE TETRACYCLINES

In 1947, chlor-tetracycline was isolated from a Missouri River (U.S.A.) mud sample by Benjamin M. Duggar. Chlor-tetracycline was the first tetracycline but Duggar's discovery has led to the isolation and subsequent development of a whole range of very powerful antibiotics, which now rank second only to the penicillins in their use world-wide.

Because they are active against a broad range of bacteria and are relatively cheap to produce, the tetracyclines quickly gained favour and are now used to treat a long list of infections. They are especially popular in developing countries because they are so inexpensive.

The extensive research done on the tetracyclines has shown them to be effective but they are also known to cause a number of toxic side-effects. The tetracyclines form calcium complexes in growing bone which may lead to life-long discoloration and enamel defects in teeth, as well as reduced bone growth. Tetracyclines also cross the placenta and have a greater toxicity in the foetus. As a result, they are prohibited in the treatment of infections in pregnant women and in children below the age of seven.

Other toxic effects include overgrowth of *Candida spp.* and *Staphylococcus spp.* in the bowel, leading to chronic infections with these organisms. Liver and kidney damage may also occur in some patients, as may allergic reactions such as hives, skin rash, asthma and contact dermatitis.

Because the tetracycline antibiotics form complexes with calcium, magnesium and iron, they should not be taken with dairy produce or any mineral and vitamin supplements containing calcium, magnesium or iron.

Table 1.1 summarises the discovery and development of the first and second generations of antibiotics during the 1940s and 1960s.

Table 1.1 Antibiotics discovered in the 1940s and 1960s

First generation of antibiotics

1942	Penicillin developed
1943	Streptomycin discovered
1945	Cephalosporins discovered
1947	Chloramphenicol discovered
1947	Chlor-tetracycline discovered

Second generation of antibiotics

1960	Methicillin developed
1961	Ampicillin developed
1963	Gentamycin developed
1964	Cephalosporins developed

Newer antibiotics

Further research took place during the 1960s, which lead to the development of the second generation of antibiotics. Among these was methicillin, a semi-synthetic derivative of penicillin, produced specifically to overcome the problem of penicillin resistance. Methicillin was hailed as a major breakthrough in the fight against bacterial resistance to penicillin and scientists believed that they could now win this battle. Unfortunately, bacteria had the last word and we now have bacteria which are resistant to methicillin.

Ampicillin is also a derivative of penicillin. It was developed to broaden the range of infections that penicillin could treat and has now replaced penicillin to a great extent. It is often the antibiotic of first choice in the treatment of a whole range of infections, including respiratory and urinary tract infections.

Amoxycillin is another widely-used penicillin derivative. Like ampicillin, it has a broad range of activity as it can treat both Gram-positive bacteria (e.g. *Streptococcus spp.* and

Staphylococcus spp.) and Gram-negative bacteria (e.g. *E. coli* and *Haemophilus influenzae*).

Gentamycin is in the same family of antibiotics as streptomycin (the anti-TB drug discovered in 1943). It is generally reserved for serious infections, as it can have severe toxic side-effects on the ears and kidneys.

THE MOST RECENT ANTIBIOTICS

Recently, a new family of antibiotics called the fluoro-quinolones has been developed by pharmaceutical laboratories. As well as being effective against a broad range of bacteria, these antibiotics can reach a high concentration in the bloodstream when taken orally. This means that many more infections, which may once have required a hospital stay, can now be treated at home.

The fluoro-quinolones are often used where long courses of antibiotics (weeks to months) are required. A whole range is now available and these are proving effective against bacteria that were once difficult to treat, such as the leprosy bacteria.

The future

The search for new and more effective drugs, which began with Florey, Chain and Selman Waksman, continues today. The pace, however, has slowed remarkably as it is now much more difficult for pharmaceutical companies to get approval for new drugs. The time delay between the discovery of an antibiotic in the laboratory and the approval to produce it commercially is so great that it has led some companies to abandon the marketplace completely.

Companies involved in the search for new antibiotics are also finding it increasingly difficult to keep up with the pace at which bacterial resistance renders them useless.

Bacterial Resistance
2   to Antibiotics

'Taking the intelligence but leaving the wisdom'

Resistance to antibiotics: is it really a problem?

Even during the early stages of antibiotic development it was clear that some bacteria could survive and multiply in the presence of antibiotics. These bacteria had acquired resistance to the effects of those antibiotics.

In an interview with the *New York Times* in 1945, Alexander Fleming warned that the misuse of penicillin could lead to the selection and multiplication of mutant forms of resistant bacteria. He also predicted that this problem of resistance would worsen if penicillin was made available in oral form, if inadequate doses were given, if a course of treatment was not completed, or if people were given too long a course of penicillin.

Just how serious is this antibiotic-resistance problem though?

MELBOURNE, AUSTRALIA

In the early 1980s, a number of hospitals in Melbourne were plagued with infections which were resistant to almost all known antibiotics. The organism causing the problem, which resulted in the deaths of a number of hospital patients, was *Staphylococcus aureus*.

This situation represents the gravest of resistance problems. It raised such fears among hospital workers that many of them wore masks at work. The bacteria were not just resistant to antibiotics, but also to antiseptics, making them virtually impossible to kill. Only one antibiotic remained effective, vancomycin, a drug which is both expensive and toxic. Doctors had no alternative but to use it. In this way, the hospital infections eventually came under control.

A close call for Melbourne. But now, we are just waiting for resistance to vancomycin to develop. When it does, we will have a very serious situation on our hands! What if resistance to vancomycin had developed in Melbourne? How would such a hospital-based infection have been treated? Would it really have become untreatable?

That was in the 1980s. Today, vancomycin resistance is indeed a reality but it occurs in a different group of bacteria —*Enterococci*. We know, however, that these bacteria are able to transfer their resistance to *Staphylococcus aureus*, the organism which causes hospital-based infections. This means it is only a question of time until resistance to vancomycin occurs in *Staphylococcus*. Then, hospital infections such as those in Melbourne really will be impossible to treat with antibiotics.

So, it is clear that we are facing a potentially disastrous situation. An infection that is untreatable by present means is now a real possibility. It's only a matter of months, or a year or two at most, according to some microbiologists.

Why do bacteria develop resistance?
Bacterial resistance to antibiotics is not a new phenomenon. In fact, it has been around for as long as bacteria themselves, but at a very low level. We can see this in soil, for example, where fungi and bacteria coexist. This coexistence is not entirely peaceful though—in fact, fungi and bacteria battle with each other for space and resources in the soil. Fungi compete with bacteria in the soil by producing antibiotics. (You may remember that many antibiotics were originally isolated from soil samples containing fungi.) In order to survive, bacteria devised a means of protecting themselves against these natural

13

antibiotics—they developed resistance. So, resistance is a natural survival mechanism.

But, if resistance to antibiotics has always been there, why has it now become so widespread? And why is it such a danger? The answers to these questions lie in the way we have approached the use of commercial antibiotics. We have over-used them in some instances and under-used them in others. We have used them inappropriately in still other circumstances. In general, we have grossly misused them and through this misuse, we have encouraged the never-ending development of resistance in bacteria.

Case History 1

Mark — Influenza

Mark was twelve years old. I had been treating him for recurrent infections of the upper respiratory tract (ear and throat infections) for almost six months. I was abroad when he developed a fever of 101 °F, a sore throat, and aches and pains. His mother brought him to the local doctor who diagnosed influenza (a viral infection) and prescribed a course of antibiotics 'just to be on the safe side'. Fortunately, Mark's mother did not fill the prescription. Instead, she sought advice from my nurse who recommended that she use anti-viral homeopathic medicine along with high-dose vitamin C. This treatment worked very well, and within forty-eight hours Mark was back to normal.

This is a good example of a case in which antibiotics clearly were not needed, because of both the diagnosis (influenza is a viral infection and should not be treated with antibiotics) and the outcome (the patient responded well to natural medicines).

Colds, 'flu, measles and herpes are examples of *viral* infections. Prescribing antibiotics to treat these infections is something I hear about frequently. Sometimes a doctor is too quick to prescribe or sometimes a patient puts pressure on the doctor to prescribe. Viral infections are *not* improved by antibiotics. They may even make the situation worse, as they can suppress the body's immune response.

In 1976 an article entitled 'What do patients know about antibiotics?' was published in the *British Journal of Medicine* (Chandler and Dugdale). Of the people questioned in this study, 55% believed that antibiotics kill viruses and only 46% believed that bacteria were killed by antibiotics. A staggering 75% believed that antibiotics should be given for colds and 'flu. Antibiotics were developed to treat bacterial infections, such as streptococcal sore throats. They should *not* be used for colds, 'flu or other viral infections.

In very simple terms, bacteria can be described as single-celled organisms. They have a cell wall, a plasma membrane and they contain genetic material. Antibiotics can kill bacteria by damaging different parts of the bacterial cell (for example, penicillin damages the cell wall).

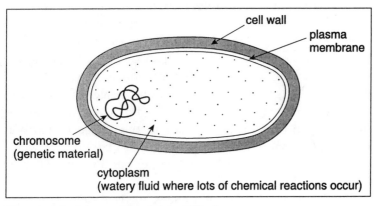

Figure 2.1 A bacterial cell (simplified)

Viruses are not living cells. They have no cell wall and no plasma membrane. They are not able to carry out chemical reactions, therefore they cannot reproduce or multiply by themselves. Since viruses do not contain structures which antibiotics can attack, these drugs are useless against viruses.

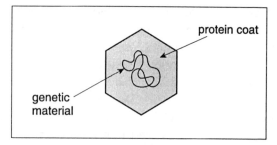

Figure 2.2 A virus (simplified)

Now you can understand why antibiotics are effective in the treatment of infections caused by bacteria, yet ineffective in the treatment of viral infections.

Case History 2

John — Recurrent sore throat and tiredness

John was the financial director of a large computer software company. He had recurring symptoms of tiredness and a sore throat, on and off for more than a year. A friend of his was a pharmacist, so to save time and money, John got antibiotics directly from his friend and treated himself. By the time he sought medical help, he had taken seven different courses of antibiotics in the space of twelve months. His symptoms were not only no better, they were now persistent, with the result that he found it very difficult to keep working.

This man was 'too busy' to seek medical help early on. Self-treatment seemed the best solution at the time. Self-medication with potentially harmful drugs only encourages the development of bacterial resistance. It can also cause long-term illness. Don't put pharmacists in the difficult position of having to diagnose and treat. The same applies to homeopathic pharmacists. Consult your doctor.

Simply by prescribing homeopathic medicines (to boost John's immune system and to undo some of the harmful effects of the antibiotics), altering his diet, as well as recommending high-dose vitamin C and live yoghurt, John's tiredness disappeared. The sore throats are now a thing of the past.

I cannot overstate how important diet is, especially for those of us living in modern cities. It is easy to end up eating a very *unnatural*, highly processed diet. Then, when the inevitable occurs and the body starts to break down, we reach for *unnatural* medicines to treat it.

It's not only doctors and patients who are at fault when it comes to over-prescribing antibiotics—pharmacists and governments are too. In many developing countries, antibiotics are freely available without a prescription. This leads to their misuse, thereby encouraging the development of resistance.

While working in Africa, I saw a situation in which drugs, sent by an aid agency to assist a particular hospital, were being sold openly in the marketplace to anyone who had the money. I have also seen cases where hospital staff have been caught stealing antibiotics which they intended to sell to the local people, as a way of boosting their income. But the problem is even more widespread than this.

ANTIBIOTIC USE IN ANIMALS

Antibiotics have been used in animal feeds for quite a long time. Farm animals, cattle and pigs in particular, are given large amounts of antibiotics as growth enhancers and to treat specific infections. These animals (and their products) end up as food in our supermarkets—either as meat or as dairy products like cheese and milk.

The bacteria in these animals tend to be multi-resistant (i.e. they have resistance to many antibiotics at the same time). This multi-resistance can be passed on to humans, through direct contact with the animals, through contaminated food, or via the soil (the faeces of these animals forms part of the soil).

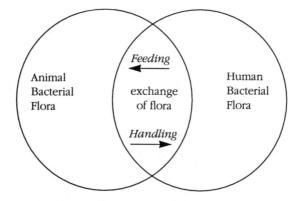

Figure 2.3 Bacterial exchange through human–animal interaction

Interactions between humans and animals can alter the bacterial flora[2] of each. Resistant bacteria can spread from the animal to the human via feeding or handling.

Many of the antibiotics approved for use in animals are being administered by farmers without veterinary supervision. One Irish farmer that I spoke to was injecting a calf with penicillin as I interviewed him. He explained to me that the calf had a sprained ankle. He was able to get a number of antibiotics from the veterinary surgeon's office without consulting the vet about the suitability of this treatment.

Over-the-counter sales of antibiotics for the farming community must be stopped. All antibiotics should be administered by a veterinary surgeon and, as with humans, should only be used as a last resort. There are many excellent homeopathic remedies available for animals. In fact, television programmes in the U.K. have reported the effectiveness of homeopathy in, for example, the treatment of mastitis in dairy cattle. The book, *A Veterinary Materia Medica* by Dr G. Mcleod, is an excellent reference for anyone wishing to try alternative treatments for a variety of conditions affecting farm animals.

It is known that small amounts of penicillin and

[2] Bacterial flora: the bacterial population which lines the skin and cavities of the body, including the respiratory and digestive tracts.

tetracycline can enhance the growth of livestock. Consequently, much greater amounts of antibiotics are given to commercial livestock as growth enhancers, rather than to treat infections. Administering even small amounts of antibiotics on a continuous basis can encourage bacterial resistance since the bacteria develop their own means of overcoming the effects of the antibiotic instead of being killed by it. So, it is easy to see why using antibiotics in this way simply helps bacteria to develop resistance.

Using penicillin and tetracycline as growth enhancers has been stopped in Europe for the most part, but not in the U.S. and other parts of the world. This is clearly an issue that must be addressed globally.

PET FOODS

One Irish study has shown that 70% of dogs have a strain of multi-resistant *E. coli*[3] in their faeces (Monaghan et al., 1981). Some of the bacteria in the bowels of these dogs were resistant to two or more antibiotics. This may well be due to the fact that antibiotics are added to commercial dog foods as growth enhancers. Even small amounts of antibiotics will encourage bacterial resistance.

Bacteria have the ability to develop resistance to almost any drug they are exposed to. This resistance is now threatening our ability to treat infections, not only in humans, but also in animals. Using antibiotics in animal feeds to enhance the growth of livestock contributes greatly to the continuation and spread of resistance. The bacteria in the bowels of commercial animals (cattle, sheep, pigs), as well as in pets (cats, dogs), are resistant not just to one or two antibiotics but to many antibiotics (multi-resistant).

Antibiotic resistance is a world-wide problem which needs the co-operation of governments, doctors, pharmacists, veterinary surgeons and farmers alike, as well as the education of the general public. It also, in my opinion, requires the full support of the World Health Organisation (WHO).

[3] E. coli is a bacterium which is a normal constituent of the bowel in most animals, including humans.

Shown below (Figure 2.4) is the hospital laboratory report of a patient suffering from a urinary tract infection. As the report shows, the bacterium responsible for this infection was *E. coli* (a common cause of urinary infections). When a laboratory isolates a bacterium, it also tests to see which antibiotics will be most effective in treating the infection.

In the report, 'S' means that the *E. coli* in the sample are *sensitive* to an antibiotic, so that antibiotic would effectively treat the infection. 'R' means that the organism is *resistant* to an antibiotic and so it would be ineffective as a treatment.

Look at the number of Rs in the report. This strain of *E. coli* is resistant to nine antibiotics—truly multi-resistant! It is only sensitive to three antibiotics, namely Netillin, Oflox and Ciproflox. Apart from being quite expensive, these drugs are rarely used to treat this condition.

Dept. of Pathology ▮▮▮▮▮▮ Hospital			Date: 03-02-95 Doctor: Dr John Mc Kenna		
Sample : Urine			Patient: ▮▮▮▮▮▮▮▮▮		
Investigation: Culture + Sensitivity					
Report : E. coli > 10^5 : Sensitivity					
Amp/Amox R	Velocef R	Augmentin R	Trimeth R	Nalidix R	Nitro R
Gentamycin R	Sulpha R	Amikacin R	Netillin S	Oflox S	Ciproflox S

Figure 2.4 Urine analysis of a patient with a urinary tract infection

A report like this, which indicates resistance to a large number of antibiotics, is very alarming. Furthermore, it is not uncommon. Soon, I expect to see strains of *E. coli* which can only be treated with one antibiotic. Not long after that there will be strains of it which are untreatable altogether.

It is interesting to note that the patient referred to above is the wife of a commercial dairy farmer. This pattern of multi-resistance is more common in patients from a farming background, probably because of the reasons mentioned earlier (i.e. the use of antibiotics in animals).

How do bacteria develop resistance?

The mechanism by which bacteria overcome antibiotics— the so-called 'magic bullets'—is fascinating. One can only be in awe of these clever and intelligent organisms and the ways in which they can outwit and conquer our efforts to kill them.

In a sense, it is our own narrow thinking and arrogance about Nature—believing that we can control Nature by killing off what we think is unnecessary or harmful—which have brought us to this deadly impasse. It is intriguing to think that we cannot control infectious diseases but that they, in fact, have the potential to control *us*. They may even wipe *us* out!

Our limited thinking and our lack of awareness of Nature are now forcing us to view things differently. We must accept that even pathogenic, disease-causing bacteria have a positive and important role to play in Nature. We don't have to understand what this role is; we need only respect it. And respect is the key to solving the problem of antibiotic resistance.

Primitive people have always had this respect. They have an understanding of the inter-connectedness of all living things and so are always attempting to work with Nature by obeying its laws. These people do not see themselves as different from or better than the rest of Nature. We, on the other hand, see humans as all-important, as separate in some way, and therefore able to rise above Nature and control it. Simple, single-celled organisms called bacteria have taught us the folly of our ways. Not only can they evade our magic bullets, they can also teach us a very valuable lesson. We all need to learn this lesson and to shift our thinking away from control—control of Nature, control of people, control of land, control of money—towards living in harmony with Nature. This is what we must learn from the so-called 'primitive peoples' whose way of life we have tried to destroy.

There will be more about our need to be in tune with Nature later. For the moment, let's examine the ways in which bacteria are able to fight back.

SPONTANEOUS MUTATIONS

Bacteria have been able to survive over the centuries through a process known as spontaneous mutation. Every so often genetic material mutates, or changes, and produces a gene which can help the bacteria to survive in the face of any toxic stuff in its environment, including antibiotics. At low levels of antibiotic usage, this is all that is necessary for their survival. The presence of an antibiotic kills off the susceptible bacteria and favours the growth of mutants which are not harmed by the antibiotic.

In the 1940s, Dr Fleming noticed these mutants in his experiments and warned about them. He predicted that the more widespread the use of antibiotics, the more widespread and more numerous these mutant forms would be. How right he was! Through spontaneous mutation the genes of bacteria can adapt, enabling them to survive in a hostile environment. This is quite clever. It shows how a change in the environment can cause unseen changes in the world of bacteria.

PLASMIDS

Ubiquitous use of antibiotics led to bacteria becoming even cleverer. They developed new, improved survival mechanisms in the form of plasmids! I first learned of plasmids in the Moyne Institute in Trinity College, Dublin, over twenty years ago. Little did I know then the importance plasmids would assume in later years, especially in my own work.

Plasmids are mini-chromosomes, or extra bits of genetic material, which occur in a bacterial cell. They are

22

independent of the chromosomes. Plasmids contain 'new' information about changes in the environment, so they help bacteria to adapt faster than ever to the changes going on around them. While we were making antibiotics widely available and patting ourselves on the back for our wonderful scientific advances, bacteria were busy developing more efficient means of protecting themselves. They were developing these mini-chromosomes, or plasmids.

Plasmids are in a constant state of change. They are continually losing genes which are of no use to the survival of the cell and, at the same time, constantly acquiring new genes. The environment dictates and selects those genes which will be of value and which need to be retained, as well as those which are no longer necessary.

Through our misuse of antibiotics, we humans have ensured the development of plasmids and their continued importance. The main function of plasmids is to prevent bacteria from being killed by antibiotics. Plasmids were unknown until the 1970s when resistance became a major problem. Plasmids rang the death knell of penicillin and warned of what was to come.

A unique characteristic of plasmids is the fact that they can be transferred from one bacterial cell to another, and from one species of bacterium to another. This is why bacteria can become resistant to a drug very quickly.

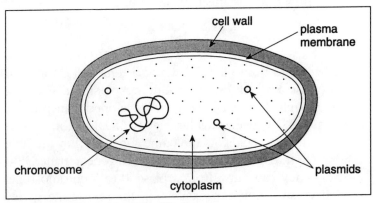

Figure 2.5 Plasmids (simplified)

JAPAN

Something very startling happened in a hospital in Japan in the late 1950s which alarmed the whole scientific community—a birth, an unusual birth, the birth of multiple drug resistance. In this hospital, a number of patients were suffering from Shigella dysentery. The bacteria causing this infection were resistant to tetracycline, the sulphonamides, streptomycin and to chloramphenicol. Multiple drug resistance was unknown prior to this. Now it suddenly sent shock waves across the world.

SOUTH AFRICA

By 1966, a number of countries had reported multiple drug resistance. In one South African hospital, 50% of the *E. coli* bacteria isolated from the faeces and urine of patients showed resistance to one or more antibiotics. This resistance information was carried by the plasmids within the bacterial cell. These plasmids were transferred to other bacteria, making them multi-resistant as well. In other words, bacteria believed in sharing their ability to defeat antibiotics with other bacteria. They don't believe in being selfish!

Drug resistance had truly become a world-wide problem. Today, virtually the whole planet has a problem, to a greater or lesser extent, with antibiotic-resistant infections. This problem is not specific to the developing or developed parts of the world—it affects us all and, in a way, unites us all.

TRANSPOSONS

There seems to be no limit to what bacteria will do in their war against antibiotics. If producing plasmids was not clever enough, bacteria have now developed transposons. Transposons are even smaller pieces of DNA (or genetic material) than plasmids. As the name suggests, they are able to jump (or transpose) from one piece of genetic material to another—they can jump from a plasmid to a chromosome, or vice versa. They can easily transfer resistance genes within a bacterial cell or from one bacterial cell to another.

24

This is an even faster and more efficient way of spreading resistance genes among a population of bacteria.

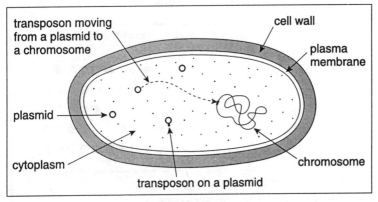

Figure 2.6 Transposons (simplified)

Spontaneous mutations, plasmids and transposons are the main methods bacteria employ to survive in the presence of antibiotics. These are the mechanisms which have led to the epidemics of bacterial resistance which currently plague many modern hospitals.

Has bacterial resistance always been there or did we create it?

To answer this question, we must visit the more remote peoples of this planet and see if they too carry bacteria that have antibiotic resistance genes.

Studies have been performed on the Bushmen tribes of Southern Africa. These people have little contact with white people, or any other people for that matter, and would never have taken antibiotics. The bacteria in stool samples from these people show very low but detectable numbers of resistant bacteria. The same result has been found in other studies of remote tribes in different parts of the world.

Among the Kalahari bushmen approximately one in fifty bacteria carry a resistance gene, whereas in European people, twenty-five out of fifty bacteria carry a resistance gene (see Figure 2.7).

So, we did not create bacterial resistance. What we have

done is encourage the development of resistant and multi-resistant bacteria. In fact, we have unwittingly allowed these bacteria to flourish and prosper.

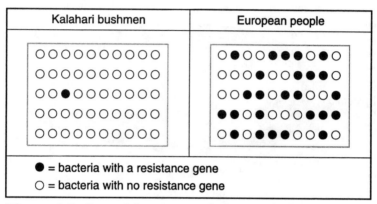

Figure 2.7 Bacterial resistance before and after antibiotic use (stool sample analysis)

Do plasmids and transposons favour bacterial survival?

Plasmids and transposons are small bits of genetic material which enable resistance genes to be acquired quickly by other bacteria. So it would seem that the answer to this question is 'yes'. However, the answer is both 'yes' and 'no'. Why?

These extra bits of genetic material allow any bacteria containing them to survive in the presence of an antibiotic; hence, survival of the species is clearly at work. But if a bacterial cell contains one or more plasmids (and/or transposons) this is disadvantageous to its survival in two ways. Firstly, carrying these extra genes (as plasmids or transposons) consumes a lot of the bacterial cell's energy, so less energy is available for its growth or reproduction. Secondly, the bacterial cell will be less virulent with these passengers. One microbiologist has described multi-resistant bacteria as 'cripples'.

So, for a bacterial cell to carry resistance genes has both advantages and disadvantages. We are constantly pressurising bacteria to carry resistance genes through our misuse of antibiotics. If this pressure is removed—by not using an antibiotic at all for a period of time—bacteria start to lose their plasmids/transposons and return to their original state.

In one hospital in Southern Africa, the doctors had a problem with resistance to an antibiotic called gentamycin. By using a less common antibiotic instead, and not using gentamycin at all for a period of five years, the particular species of bacteria (*Klebsiella pneumonia* which can cause lung infections) lost its resistance genes and once again became sensitive to gentamycin. Gentamycin therefore became useful again.

It is good to know this. It suggests that a more prudent approach to the use of antibiotics will indeed result in bacterial changes. These changes will lead to reduced bacterial resistance and a return to the natural state of susceptibility to antibiotics. This is a beautiful example of the balances that work within Nature.

The consequences of resistance

As with all situations in life, we can choose to view things negatively or positively. The negative way of viewing resistance is evident in certain literature, particularly from the U.S., and when listening to some doctors being interviewed on American television. The problem of resistance is portrayed as a plague which can wipe out the whole of humanity in a short space of time. This may not be untrue, but if we created the problem, we can surely solve it too.

The more positive way of viewing resistance is to see it as a blessing in disguise. It is a blessing because it makes us stop and think. It makes us become more responsible for our actions (for example, not using an antibiotic as a quick fix if you have a cough or a cold). It is forcing all of us to educate ourselves not just about antibiotics but about the harmful effects of all drugs. It is asking us to make choices about our lifestyles. In more subtle ways, this problem of resistance is challenging our view of ourselves and our world, since we are finding it harder to view ourselves as wiser or more knowledgeable than single-celled bacteria or as separate from them. It challenges our concept of control, not just of Nature but of many things in our lives.

Control of anything or anyone never works. When we glimpse the beauty at work within bacteria, humans and the whole of Nature, we begin to realise that control prevents this beauty from showing itself. Resistance challenges us to be more in tune with Nature and with ourselves, so resistance is making us more aware!

In the previous chapter, you saw a hospital laboratory analysis of a urine sample. It showed that the strain of *E. coli* present in the sample was resistant to most antibiotics. I treated this patient with cranberry juice (shown in a number of studies to be effective in the treatment of urinary tract infections), a complex homeopathic remedy containing Echinacea in ampoule form, and high-dose vitamin C. A repeat urine culture two weeks later showed no growth of *E. coli*. The infection had responded.

Summary
Resistance to antibiotics is a major public health problem. It is threatening our ability to fight even common infections like tonsillitis, ear infections and urinary tract infections.

Because it is such a massive problem, global in its dimensions and not well understood by the public, an organisation called the Alliance for the Prudent Use of Antibiotics has been established in the U.S. to address the issue. The main aims of this organisation are to encourage people to take a more responsible approach to the use of antibiotics, and to promote improved use of antibiotics through communication of research information from different countries around the world. It also seeks to educate people—doctors, patients, veterinary surgeons, farmers, pharmacists, pharmaceutical companies and lay people alike. This kind of international co-operation involving all those interested in the use of antibiotics is absolutely necessary.

3

The Use and Abuse of Antibiotics

'The blind leading the blind'

Antibiotics have been in use for nearly fifty years, although it is only more recently that they have been in mass production. What did we do before the advent of antibiotics? This knowledge will be vital to our survival in years to come, as an increasing number of common infections such as tonsillitis, middle ear infections and urinary tract infections, become untreatable with antibiotics.

For simplicity, I have used 1940 as the dividing line between the pre-antibiotic and the antibiotic eras. Prior to 1940, there were no antibiotics. How did parents handle simple infections in their children? How did doctors treat more serious infections?

A common-sense approach was obviously being used— do little to treat the infection initially, allow the body to fight it naturally and in so doing, build up one's natural resistance to it. Only when the body was clearly not winning the battle was intervention required.

In general, people depended on herbal medicines and folk cures. Ireland had a strong tradition of herbal medicine, with a doctor or herbalist ready to help in the treatment of infections. As in many other cultures, the knowledge of growing and using herbal medicines was handed down from generation to generation. Doctors depended to a great extent on natural substances such as iron, mercury and antimony. In Germany, there was a tradition in homeopathic medicine.

Many doctors were trained in the art of homeopathy and indeed, there were a number of lay homeopaths as well.

From the mid-1800s until the turn of the century, homeopathic medicine was extremely popular in Europe and North America. In the early 1900s though, the American Medical Association (AMA) secured a strong political lobby to close many homeopathic colleges and hospitals. By 1920, the number of these hospitals had dropped to a mere seven.

The rise of conventional medicine was linked to the rise of the pharmaceutical companies. The AMA had found a powerful ally, which may explain their considerable political clout. It may also explain why most medical research is sponsored by pharmaceutical companies and why medical students are taught pharmacology (the use of drugs) as the primary means of treating patients.

It was in 1928 that Alexander Fleming made his now-famous discovery which led to the production of penicillin. Fleming showed that a mould called *Penicillium notatum* arrested the growth of certain bacteria (*Staphylococcus spp.* and *Streptococcus spp.*). Nothing much happened to this piece of research for 17 years.

In 1935, a German researcher showed that a dye called Prontosil Red cured mice that were infected with *Streptococcus spp.* (the bacteria that can cause sore throats). Prontosil Red was the precursor of a group of antibiotic-like drugs called sulphonamides (or sulpha drugs). These drugs are still in use today. Septrin, for example, which contains sulphamethoxazole, is used to treat respiratory and urinary infections.

It wasn't until 1945 that Florey and Chain continued the research started by Fleming. They purified penicillin and concentrated it for clinical use. They also demonstrated the effectiveness of penicillin against a whole range of bacterial infections including diphtheria, tetanus and anthrax. As a direct result of this work, antibiotics were put into clinical use and developed for mass production. When the chemical formula of penicillin was eventually identified, chemists and biochemists were able to synthesise antibiotics in the laboratory. Consequently, many of the antibiotics in use today come from this source.

Pre-1940, the treatment of common infections depended on:
- *Herbs*
- *Homeopathy*
- *Traditional/Folk cures*
- *Common sense*

In the post-1940, or antibiotic, era there was a gradual decrease in people's reliance on natural medicines and an increased dependence on drugs, including antibiotics. Today, this dependence has become so strong that it can render some people helpless when faced with a sick child, for example. It is only now that we are beginning to see the folly of our ways, with the general public starting to express an increased desire to relearn the old methods.

Post-1940, the treatment of common infections showed:
- *A decreased reliance on folk cures, common sense, herbs and homeopathy*
- *An increased reliance on sulpha drugs and antibiotics*

Antibiotics are now being rendered useless

Antibiotics are potentially life-saving drugs. They represent a wonderful advancement in medical science. When they first came on the scene, we all believed that the scourge of infectious disease would be gone forever and that humankind could live in a virtually infection-free world.

The truth has turned out to be rather different. Antibiotics are now being rendered useless by the very bacteria they were intended to destroy. Bacterial resistance is developing at an alarming rate, to the point where many hospital-based doctors are deeply concerned about the future.

Recently, I heard a group of doctors in New York speak about the new epidemic of tuberculosis (TB) that is occurring in the U.S. They were saying that this latest outbreak of TB is proving extremely difficult to treat because the bacterium that causes it (*Mycobacterium tuberculosis*), is now multi-resistant to most of the standard drugs. Patients with this form of TB are untreatable at present. Doctors throughout Europe have also warned about the alarming increase in bacterial resistance to antibiotics and have urged general practitioners to be much more cautious in the way in which they prescribe. You, as a potential patient, can assist your GP by discussing the alternatives with him/her and by asking for natural medicines.

The truth of the matter, however, is that antibiotics have become a major public health hazard and, in the very near future, common infections may not respond to antibiotic treatment at all. Because of this overuse and abuse of antibiotics, we have lost sight of the fact that Nature has its own methods of fighting back, i.e. in producing multi-resistant strains of bacteria. Ironically, it is to Nature and natural medicine that we must look for a way out of this predicament. In this book, I want to show that there are effective methods of treating infections which are not only free of side-effects, but are also less likely to result in bacterial resistance in the years to come.

The dangers of excessive antibiotic use
RESISTANCE
If antibiotics such as penicillin are used inappropriately, or for too short a period of time, bacteria can develop resistance. These resistant strains are then able to counteract the effects of penicillin when they next come into contact with this antibiotic. In this way, the drug starts to become ineffective. When many different types of bacteria start to develop resistance to penicillin, the drug starts to become useless. As a result, more powerful antibiotics have to be synthesised and manufactured. However, the pace at which bacterial resistance is developing is much faster than the pace at which drug companies can produce new antibiotics.

ALLERGIC REACTIONS
Because of the overuse of antibiotics, allergies are increasingly common. These allergic reactions can vary from

a nettle-sting-type skin rash to oedema (tissue swelling), bronchospasm (constriction of the airways) and shock.

Antibiotics such as tetracycline and amoxycillin can disturb the intestinal bacteria, especially the 'good', healthy bacteria like *Lactobacillus acidophilus* and *Bifidobacterium bifidus*. This can lead to intestinal problems such as diarrhoea, flatulence and abdominal distension (bloating). There is now evidence to suggest that disturbances of the intestinal bacteria may be important in the development of bowel disorders such as ulcerative colitis and cancer of the colon.

Another problem that can result is the overgrowth of yeast and fungi in the bowel, leading to intestinal candidiasis. This is now a major problem in the western world and coincides with the overuse of antibiotics. Candidiasis used to be a disease seen only in people whose immunity was compromised—for example, in babies whose immunity is still developing, in the elderly whose immunity is in decline, and in patients whose immunity has been suppressed for some reason (e.g. being on long-term steroids). In the 1990s, intestinal candidiasis is affecting all age groups and all types of people. This concerns me as it suggests that people's immunity is under threat.

Case History 3

Sarah — Abdominal pain and loss of appetite

Sarah, a six-year-old girl, had been suffering from a pain in her tummy (abdominal pain) and loss of appetite for three months. Prior to the onset of these symptoms, she had received four courses of antibiotics for ear infections which were very resistant to treatment. I diagnosed her as having intestinal dysbiosis (a disturbance in the bacterial population of the bowel). I altered her diet to exclude sugar and processed foods, and to include live yoghurt and whey. I also gave her appropriate homeopathic remedies. Not only did her abdominal pain disappear and her appetite improve, but her ear infections disappeared as well.

This case is typical of many children who have been given one or more courses of antibiotics, especially broad spectrum antibiotics[4] (e.g. tetracycline and amoxycillin). Antibiotics can disturb the 'good' bacteria which line the digestive tract. These bacteria manufacture a number of vitamins which the body needs for good health.

Antibiotics may also have a suppressive effect on the immune system. Certain antibiotics, including tetracycline and the sulphonamides, can inhibit the activity of the white blood cells which engulf and destroy bacteria. Other antibiotics are known to inhibit antibody production, thus lowering immunity (Hauser and Remington, 1982). Antibiotics have also been shown to increase the likelihood of recurrent infections. Studies published in 1974 (Diamont and Diamont), and more recently in 1991 (Cantekin et al.), have shown that children with ear-aches who received antibiotics, especially in the first few days, were much more likely to develop recurrent ear problems than those in whom treatment was delayed or to whom a placebo was given. In conventional medical circles, it is now widely accepted that doctors should either delay treatment of ear-aches or not treat them at all.

This documentation supports other evidence which shows that antibiotics can indeed suppress one's natural immune response to an infection and can set up a situation in which the infection recurs.

Specific problems with certain antibiotics
Chloramphenicol
It is not uncommon for this drug to cause a reduction in the white blood cell count, particularly the type of white cell that fights against bacteria invading the body (granulocytes). In rare cases, approximately one in 100,000, it can cause death by suppressing bone marrow function. This is why it has been taken off the market in Europe and North America, although it is still being used in many African countries.

---

[4] A broad spectrum antibiotic is one which can kill a wide range of bacteria. A narrow spectrum antibiotic is much more specific and generally targets one type of bacterium.

Tetracyclines

Tetracyclines are sold under various trade names—achromycin, chymocyclar, deteclo, hostacycline, imperacin, mysteclin, tetrabid, tetrachel, and tetrex. They can damage the growing bones and teeth of the foetus and young children below the age of seven. Tetracyclines are absorbed by bones and teeth because the drug binds calcium phosphate. This damages the dental enamel of the tooth with pitting, as well as causing yellow/brown discoloration of the teeth and increasing susceptibility to dental cavities.

Tetracyclines are known to decrease the levels of some of the B vitamins in the body by disturbing their absorption in the bowel. They can also disturb the bacterial flora of the bowel. In addition, tetracyclines can cause diarrhoea, especially with prolonged use. Less commonly, they can increase the pressure around the brain in a condition called benign intra-cranial hypertension.

The tetracyclines are potentially quite damaging antibiotics. They are often prescribed for the long-term treatment of teenage acne and are used for three to six, and in some cases twelve, months. It worries me that people are taking this type of antibiotic for such long periods of time.

Aminoglycosides

Included in this group of antibiotics is the anti-TB drug, streptomycin, as well as gentamycin, kanamycin, tobramycin, neomycin and amikacin. They are commonly used to treat infections where the invading bacteria cause urinary tract infections, peritonitis, and wound infections after bowel surgery. This particular group of antibiotics is quite toxic as they can cause damage to the auditory nerve and so lead to deafness. They are also capable of damaging the kidneys as well as causing skin rashes and drug-induced fevers.

Sulphonamides

The sulphonamides can cause some serious side-effects, including allergic reactions of many kinds (skin rash, fever, hepatitis, low white cell count, purpuric rash, aplastic anaemia), diarrhoea and the formation of crystals in the urine. Sulphonamides are also known to cause pancreatitis and diabetes mellitus.

Less serious side-effects include malaise, headache, nausea and vomiting, but these are usually transient. The sulphonamides are sold under the trade names of septrin, bactrim, antrimox, cotrimel, chemotrim and tricomox.

Antibiotic abuse — the reasons why

It is vitally important that we understand the mistakes we have made in the past with antibiotics so that they will not be repeated in the future. We need to be aware of where we have gone wrong and why?

Antibiotics are often prescribed for viral infections such as colds, 'flu, glandular fever, herpes infections and gastro-enteritis. As stated in the previous chapter, antibiotics have no role to play in viral infections as they neither kill nor stop the multiplication of viruses. Sometimes a viral infection can weaken the immune system, particularly in certain 'at risk' groups like the elderly, the very young, post-surgery or other trauma patients. As a result, a viral infection may sometimes lead to a secondary bacterial infection and this is often the reason why an antibiotic is prescribed for viral infections. Surely it would make more sense to wait and see if a bacterial infection develops and, if concerned, to boost the immunity of the person at risk to prevent a secondary bacterial infection developing.

Antibiotics are also prescribed for relatively minor infections instead of using simpler methods. Very often an infection requires no treatment at all, as your body will naturally fight it. But, if necessary, this fight can be assisted by natural means. It is important to let your body fight an infection, since this will allow you to build up a natural resistance to that particular infection. Only when the body is clearly not winning the battle should one intervene. Remember also that many antibiotics do not kill bacteria outright as is commonly believed, but rather they only stop their growth. Your immune system must do the rest.

Antibiotics should be used as the last resort, not the first.

This book will describe methods which can be used in the initial stages of infection. If these measures fail, there may then be a role for antibiotics. In this way, antibiotics will become the exception rather than the rule and bacterial resistance will become less of a problem.

What if an antibiotic must be used?
There are a number of steps you can take to offset the negative effects an antibiotic may cause as well as maximising the effectiveness of the antibiotic:

• Take live yoghurt or other bacterial supplements, such as Acidophilus capsules, with the antibiotic to prevent damage to the intestinal bacteria which are important for a healthy bowel.

• Use an immune booster to assist your body's immune response to the infection as there is some evidence which suggests that antibiotics can suppress different parts of the immune system. (Substances that boost immunity are discussed in Chapter 6.)

• Take vitamin C along with an antibiotic as vitamin C is known to increase the blood levels of certain antibiotics, thus making them more effective. I recommend a dose of 2000–3000 mg daily.

• Take the antibiotic for the prescribed period as stopping before the course has been completed will encourage the development of bacterial resistance and make a recurrence of the disease more difficult to treat.

• Insist on knowing all the side-effects before agreeing to use an antibiotic. Your doctor or pharmacist should be able to assist you in this regard.

Case History 4

Gerard — Recurrent ear and chest infections

Gerard was seven years old and was suffering from recurrent ear and chest infections when his mother brought him to see me. His doctor had treated him with antibiotics each time he had an ear-ache or a chest infection. His mother handed me a list of the antibiotics used and the dates when they were prescribed. (Always keep a record of drugs that you have been prescribed and the dates, as Gerard's mother did.) Here is the list.

Date	Prescription
11/02/1993	Distaclor
18/03/1993	Erythroped
17/05/1993	Augmentin
30/05/1993	Septrin
10/06/1993	Distaclor
10/07/1993	Septrin
15/07/1993	Augmentin
01/09/1993	Augmentin
10/09/1993	Augmentin
27/09/1993	Distaclor
23/12/1993	Augmentin
04/01/1994	Septrin
24/02/1994	Erythroped
27/02/1994	Distaclor

This makes fourteen antibiotics given to a young child within a twelve-month period. This is frightening, but not the worst case I've seen. When I sent Gerard for testing, he had gross disturbance of his bacterial flora as well as pancreatic damage. A change in diet, homeopathic medicines to boost his immunity, high-dose vitamin C and live yoghurt helped this child enormously. Since coming to see me, he has not needed another antibiotic and the infections have ceased. This is the beauty of natural medicine. It is possible to help so many people by getting them off conventional drugs and using safe medicines.

Gerard's case history illustrates a prescribing pattern that is doing immense damage, not only to patients who have to suffer the side-effects of these drugs, but also to the medical profession whose credibility is being undermined. That such a quantity of drugs can be prescribed to a young child is shocking and it clearly highlights the futility of continuing to educate doctors in drug therapy alone. It is imperative that they be trained in the use of natural medicines. Interestingly, most medical students and doctors would favour such training. With your help, it can happen.

Conventional and Alternative Medical 4 Approaches

'The scientific and the intuitive meet'

The conventional medical approach to treating infections

Conventional medicine is very much disease-oriented, almost to the point of viewing the disease as separate from the patient. As a consequence of this, infections are approached from a curative point of view—drugs which kill the bacterium or fungus are used to cure you of the disease. So, if two patients present with the same infection, such as a streptococcal sore throat, they will receive the same treatment.

This curative, or anti-microbial, approach to treating an infection seldom looks at the reasons why the infection has arisen in the first place. Finding these reasons is of vital importance when it comes to prevention. The underlying reasons why infections occur, and particularly when they recur, may be related to a weakened immune system in one patient, to poor nutrition in another, and to emotional stress or trauma in yet another. The conventional approach will use an antibiotic to treat not just the initial infection but all infections thereafter. If one antibiotic does not work, others will be tried.

Despite the side-effects associated with these drugs, courses of antibiotics are readily and frequently prescribed. This illustrates a fundamental weakness in medical training, with doctors only being taught this particular approach to treating infections. Many GPs are caught in this trap. Their training has focused on the use of drugs but many of them feel increasingly uncomfortable with this drug-based approach and are looking for alternatives. You can help your doctor by encouraging him/her to find these alternatives.

Because the conventional approach is mainly curative and not preventative, and because it has side-effects, many patients come to me, knowing that I am committed to a safer and more natural form of medicine.

The conventional medical approach
- *is curative*
- *is not holistic; it does not look for the underlying cause*
- *has side-effects*

The alternative medical approach to treating infections

Alternative medicine is more patient-oriented and views the patient in much broader terms. It takes account of the fact that you are not just a physical body, but that you have a mind or mental body as well (with a particular set of thought patterns which affect the way you view everything around you). It recognises that you have an emotional body which has a strong interaction with your physical body (e.g. anger raises your blood pressure significantly), and a soul or spiritual body which is the very core of your being. Any form of medicine which recognises and treats these different levels of being facilitates a better understanding of the origins of many illnesses and of us as people. A very good example of interaction between mind and body is discussed in Chapter 10, which deals with stress.

Since it is very broad in its approach, alternative medicine is able to be both curative *and* preventative. This approach could even be regarded as being more preventative than curative because it looks beyond the patient's symptoms—it looks for the underlying causes of an infection. As a result, it is often better able to prevent the recurrence of an illness. Treatment with natural immune-enhancing medicines, certain homeopathic medicines, and vitamin/mineral supplements helps to ensure that an illness does not recur in the future.

This approach educates patients and gives them more control over their own health. It also breaks the vicious cycle of becoming dependent on one antibiotic after another. Because these alternative medicines are natural, they are also for the most part free of side-effects. (The issue of side-effects is discussed in each section of the book.)

The alternative medical approach
* *is both curative and preventative*
* *is holistic*
* *has few or no side-effects*

Although these two approaches are quite different, they share the same aim—to help you, the patient. If both conventional and alternative practitioners can keep the patient in the foreground and their own vested interests in the background, we shall all benefit. Conventional doctors can learn from alternative practitioners, while the latter can benefit from the medical research, the laboratory investigations and the access to emergency back-up services of conventional medicine.

Open-mindedness and a willingness to respect another approach to healing is the way forward. I personally feel that neither approach is inherently wrong. Both have much to offer a patient and each other. I feel the future in medicine lies in incorporating both forms of medicine into a system of healing where the intuitive ability of a healer is developed alongside his/her scientific skills. The art of healing must combine with the science of medicine to create a future.

Childhood Infections

'Antibiotics — the exception, not the rule'

Each year in the U.S. over $500 million worth of antibiotics are prescribed to treat one single problem—ear-ache in young children. The prescribing of antibiotics for childhood infections has risen alarmingly over the past twenty years. Reread the case history in the Preface just to remind yourself of how children are being treated. This excessively heavy prescribing of antibiotics costs a great deal, not only financially but also in human terms.

In this chapter, you will learn that most infections in children are viral and so do not require antibiotics. I shall deal only with the more common childhood infections including those of the upper respiratory tract, the lower respiratory tract, the intestine and the urinary tract. I shall also point out situations where an antibiotic *may* be required but please remember that most childhood infections *do not* require an antibiotic.

Upper respiratory tract infections
(NASAL, SINUS, THROAT AND EAR INFECTIONS)
Fifty per cent of all infections in children are respiratory by nature. Upper respiratory tract infections such as colds, 'flu and snotty noses are viral so antibiotics have no part to play in their treatment. Even if the discharge from the nostrils is yellowish or greenish, swabs consistently show no bacterial growth. If in doubt, have a nasal swab done by your family doctor as this will show whether the infection is bacterial or

not. The majority of nasal infections, however, are viral and they respond well to anti-viral treatment.

Anti-viral measures include a specific homeopathic remedy and enhancement of the immune system, as well as vitamin C and, in some cases, zinc. (You will learn more about anti-viral measures in Chapters 6 and 7, which deal with herbal medicine and homeopathy.)

Children who do not respond to anti-viral measures usually have an allergy or intolerance to one or more foods, most commonly dairy produce or sugar which are mucus-forming foods. If an allergy or intolerance to a specific food is suspected, it is essential to avoid it during treatment.

There are two situations which sometimes warrant the use of an antibiotic. The first of these is acute *otitis media* or middle ear infection. Somewhere between 30–50% of these infections (the literature seems to vary as to the exact percentage) are bacterial, most commonly caused by *Streptococcus pneumoniae*. The other situation which may require an antibiotic is a bacterial sore throat, which is most commonly caused by *haemolytic-streptococci*. However, only about 30% of throat infections are bacterial. If your doctor prescribes an antibiotic for an ear or throat infection, make sure to use an immune stimulant along with it (Chapter 6) and live yoghurt to protect the intestinal flora (Chapter 8). Some studies have shown that taking vitamin C along with an antibiotic can enhance the activity of the antibiotic, thus making it more effective. Furthermore, the duration of antibiotic treatment can be shortened as a result of this enhanced activity, thereby reducing the side-effects. This is clearly an area which needs further research.

With middle ear infections, the recommendation is to wait a few days before taking an antibiotic and in many cases to use no antibiotic at all. Scientists have recently established a link between an allergy to dairy products and recurrent ear infections, so this possibility should be checked before using an antibiotic (Schmidt, 1990).

Researchers have also shown that many of the children being prescribed antibiotics for ear-ache actually have no bacterial infection in the middle ear. Other possible causes of ear-ache include: a viral infection; a blockage of the Eustachian tube (this tube connects the throat and middle ear and can get blocked by throat infections); or an infection of the lining of the ear canal. The diagnosis of a middle ear infection is based on the presence of ear pain associated with fever. Upon examination, the ear drum appears red and bulging. Infants too young to complain of ear-ache are usually irritable and restless. The pain may be so severe that they scream.

If an antibiotic is necessary, studies have shown that short courses of treatment are just as effective as longer ones. For example, two-, four- and five-day courses are equally as effective as a ten-day course. In addition, delaying treatment for a day or two and using only pain killers will show if an antibiotic is really necessary.

Using antibiotics in the treatment of ear-ache can predispose to recurrent ear infections, especially with multi-resistant bacteria. For example, children treated with amoxycillin have been shown to be two to eight times more likely to get a recurrent infection.

- *Most upper respiratory tract infections are viral. Approximately 30–50% of* otitis media *and about 30% of sore throats are bacterial. These are two situations in which an antibiotic may be necessary.*
- *If it is necessary to use an antibiotic for a middle ear infection or a sore throat, take both an immune booster and live yoghurt with it. Vitamin C can also enhance the activity of the antibiotic.*

Lower respiratory tract infections
(CHEST INFECTIONS)
As in upper respiratory tract infections, antibiotics have a very limited role to play in the treatment of lower respiratory tract infections.

CROUP
With croup, 95% of infections are viral (usually caused by the para-influenza group of viruses) and anti-viral measures

should therefore be used. It is important to discuss the other 5% of cases, however, as they tend to be bacterial (*Haemophilus influenzae*). These infections, which usually make the child much more ill and toxic, can be life-threatening. If there is any suspicion that croup is bacterial (the warning signs are in Table 5.1), the child should be admitted to hospital. In general though, the treatment of croup with an antibiotic 'in case of a bacterial infection' is bad medicine since 95% of the time there will be no need for an antibiotic.

Table 5.1 Signs of bacterial croup

1. The child is very unwell and toxic (not the case in viral croup)
2. The child may have a muffled voice
3. The child cannot swallow saliva and drools

BRONCHITIS

Unlike adults, the majority of acute bronchitis infections in children are viral. A number of different viruses may be responsible for the infection including respiratory syncytial virus, para-influenza virus, adenovirus or rhinovirus. Again, anti-viral treatment is what's needed here.

Childhood bronchitis is very rarely bacterial. When it is, the infection is more serious and would most commonly be caused by *Streptococcus pneumoniae*. With the majority of cases of acute bronchitis in children, antibiotics have no role to play. Only in cases where there are definite signs of a serious lower respiratory tract infection (see Table 5.2) should an antibiotic be considered. If there are signs of a bacterial infection, some doctors admit the child to hospital, which is probably the safer option; others prefer to treat the child at home.

Although *Streptococcus pneumoniae* is usually responsible, it is important to consider the possibility of staphylococcal pneumonia as this requires a rather different course of treatment—in conventional medicine, cloxacillin or flucloxacillin are the antibiotics of choice. Most deaths due to childhood pneumonia are caused by *Staphylococcus spp.* and most of these children were not prescribed the antibiotics cloxacillin or flucloxacillin. Pneumonia which is caused by other bacteria is very rare, except in those whose immunity is compromised.

In cases of bacterial pneumonia, antibiotics have a definite role to play. I recommend taking high-dose vitamin C for the duration of the course of treatment.

Table 5.2 Signs of a serious lower respiratory tract infection

---

1. Rate of breathing increases to
   — over 60 breaths per minute in infants
   — over 40 breaths per minute in toddlers
   — over 30 breaths per minute in school children
2. Respiratory distress (i.e. gasping for air)
3. Cyanosis (i.e. turning blue)
4. Pulse increases to
   — over 180 beats per minute in infants
   — over 160 beats per minute in toddlers
   — over 110 beats per minute in school children

• *Most cases of acute bronchitis in children are viral; rarely are they bacterial.* Streptococcus pneumoniae *is the bacterium most commonly responsible for bacterial infections. Watch for signs of a serious lower respiratory tract infection.*

CASE HISTORY 5

Seán — Persistent cough

Seán had a persistent cough for more than three years. This four-year-old child developed the cough at the age of six months, shortly after vaccination with the 3-in-1 vaccine (diphtheria, tetanus and whopping cough). The cough was dry, came in bouts, got worse at night and occasionally changed to a productive cough with yellow sputum. All investigations (chest X-ray, blood tests, sputum culture and swabs) were negative. The child's diet was well-balanced and very healthy.

I treated this as a viral infection following vaccination and used an anti-viral homeopathic medicine, high-dose vitamin C and an immune enhancer. The cough, which had been present for 3½ years, began to improve and was gone within two weeks.

Seán's cough was due to a viral infection of the lower respiratory tract and it responded very well to anti-viral treatment. The fact that it began just after vaccination was interesting because I have seen many children react negatively to certain vaccines, particularly the pertussis (whooping cough) and the measles vaccines. In some children, these vaccines appear to suppress the immune system and allow a chronic infection to develop, as in Seán's case. In situations like these, I recommend homeopathic vaccination.

It is not uncommon for vaccines to cause difficulties, especially the 3-in-1 and the MMR vaccines. This is why many parents opt for the 2-in-1 vaccine which excludes the whooping cough vaccine.

This case exemplifies the fact that it is relatively easy to treat chronic (or acute) viral infections in young children. When a child does not respond, I refer him or her for testing to see if other factors are involved in the infection—allergies, reactions to medicines or vaccines, poor nutrition, exposure to various pollutants including heavy metals, parasites, less common infections including tuberculosis and so on. By doing thorough testing, using both conventional and alternative medical techniques, I have been able to find the underlying cause in all cases. This is so much better than treating the patient blindly, time and time again, in the hope that something will work. It does not make sense to keep a child on medication long-term. I believe it is much more fruitful to put time and effort into finding the underlying cause and to treat that.

There is very little basis for using antibiotics with patients who have wheezy bronchitis or asthma, since they are both caused by viruses. As with acute bronchitis, the viruses responsible are respiratory syncytial virus, rhinovirus and para-influenza virus. Anti-viral treatment is called for, not antibiotics. Only rarely is wheezy bronchitis a bacterial infection. When it is, the organism concerned is usually *Streptococcus pneumoniae.*

RECURRENT RESPIRATORY INFECTIONS
Some children get recurrent upper or lower respiratory tract infections, or a mixture of the two. These are *always* viral. In some cases, they can be aggravated by environmental factors —stress, a smoky atmosphere, a damp house. There is no basis for the use of antibiotics—anti-viral measures should be used.

THE CHILD WHO DOES NOT GET BETTER
In addition to infective causes, there may be other reasons why a child does not respond to treatment, either with conventional drugs, alternative medicine, or both. Below are five conditions worth keeping in mind.

1. Tuberculosis
The child is often free of symptoms and the disease is picked up only when a chest X-ray is performed. It may be associated with weight loss. Tuberculosis is not very common in Europe.

2. Cystic fibrosis
Cystic fibrosis is a relatively rare condition affecting approximately 1 in 2000 children. It may be associated with failure to thrive, loose stools and prolapse of the rectum. The majority of patients are diagnosed in infancy, but a significant number with mild symptoms are first diagnosed in later childhood. The diagnosis is made by finding high sodium and chloride levels in sweat.

3. Mycoplasma pneumonia

This affects older children, of school-going age (5–15 years), and can cause a wide range of respiratory tract infections. These children produce a clinical picture of lassitude, loss of appetite and a cough that is hard to get rid of. There may be a fever and a sore throat as well. The diagnosis is often suspected from the chest X-ray and is confirmed by finding specific antibodies in the bloodstream.

4. Reduced IGA

IGA is an antibody that protects the lining of the respiratory tract. Children with impaired immunity (i.e. reduced IGA) fail to thrive and show a pattern of loose stools. A blood test is sufficient to diagnose this condition. It is much rarer than any of the above.

5. Inhalation of a foreign body (e.g. a peanut or wheel of a toy car)

Sometimes a child can inhale a small object into the airway. Babies and toddlers are most at risk, as they tend to put everything in their mouths. The foreign body may block the airway at any level. If it lodges in the lower airway, there will be no symptoms for a time until part of the lung collapses or an infection develops. If this is suspected as the reason why a cough, for example, is unresponsive to treatment, chest X-rays, including X-rays from the side (lateral chest X-rays) should be carried out. However, translucent objects such as a sweet may not show up on an X-ray and bronchoscopy (passing a scope down the airway to have a look) may be necessary.

Conditions 1–4 above are best treated with a combination of conventional and alternative medicines. In all of these cases testing would be important in order to assess which medicines to use, what dosage to give and how long the treatment period should be. Treatment should involve the co-operation of a paediatrician (a specialist in childhood diseases) and a homeopathic doctor. The fifth condition, inhalation of a foreign body, should be treated in hospital.

Infections of other parts of the body

GASTRO-ENTERITIS

Like most respiratory infections, 60% of cases of gastro-enteritis in children under the age of five, are caused by a virus. It is uncommon for bacteria to be responsible. But even if the infection is suspected of being bacterial, antibiotics may be the *wrong* form of treatment. In gastro-enteritis, antibiotics can exacerbate the condition by worsening the diarrhoea. They can also predispose the child to a super-infection with *Candida spp.* or *Staphylococcus spp.*, both of which may be life-threatening. If bacterial infection is suspected, stool cultures should be done. The mainstay of treatment must always be rehydration, either orally or intravenously.

• *Most cases of gastro-enteritis are viral. Even if they are bacterial, one should be very careful about using antibiotics.*

URINARY TRACT INFECTIONS

In contrast to most respiratory and bowel infections, urinary tract infections (UTIs) are generally bacterial in nature. This means that antibiotics may have a role to play in their treatment. However, it is always better to use natural methods first. I have successfully treated many cases of UTI using only natural medicines. The case mentioned in Chapter 3 (p.28), in which I used natural methods including cranberry juice to treat a UTI, shows that in many instances antibiotics are not necessary. If natural methods do not control the infection, then there is a place for antibiotics.

UTIs are commonly caused by organisms derived from the bowel. The cause of the infection is usually contamination of the vagina or urethra with faeces from the bowel, thereby allowing the bacteria in the bowel access to the urinary tract.

The most common bacterium in urinary tract infections is *Escherichia coli* (*E. coli*). All children under the age of five years who have recurrent urinary tract infections should have an IVP (intravenous pyelogram) done. This involves injecting dye into one of the veins in the arm and taking X-rays of the urinary tract to screen for abnormalities. The most common abnormality detected is reflux of urine from the bladder back up into the ureter.

• *Most urinary tract infections are bacterial and so antibiotics may have a role to play. However, use a natural medicine first.*

Summary
Most common childhood infections are *viral*. Whether discussing upper respiratory tract, lower respiratory tract or bowel infections, the mainstay of treatment should be anti-viral, *not antibiotics*!

For the treatment of viral infections:
• Boost the immune system—Chapter 6 will describe how this can be done.
• Take vitamin C—dosage and usage are discussed in Chapter 9, which deals with nutritional supplements.
• Use anti-viral homeopathic medicines—these are discussed in Chapter 7.

There are, however, a few situations which sometimes require an antibiotic. These include:
• a sore throat with a yellowish exudate on the tonsil—30% of these cases are bacterial.
• middle ear infections—30–50% of these cases are bacterial. Wait to use antibiotics. Use natural medicines first.
• urinary tract infections—use natural medicines first.

This chapter has dealt only with the more common infections in children. I hope it has clarified the position regarding the need to use antibiotics and illustrates the point that *most infections do not require an antibiotic.*

We live in a quick-fix, superficial society. We do not want to tolerate any pain or suffering, we want instant cures. The price of not truly treating the cause of the pain or illness is acceptable, provided we don't have to suffer. The medical profession supports this attitude by prescribing pills to take away the illness—or so it would appear. I see so many children with recurrent infections in whom the illness clearly is not being treated. A quick-fix is being provided over and over again. No one benefits from such a short-term, blinkered approach—the child does not get better, the parent becomes more anxious and the doctor becomes increasingly frustrated as there is a limit to the number of drugs which he/she can prescribe. Furthermore, society in general suffers, as the problem of bacterial resistance continues to grow because of these prescribing practices.

The days of using antibiotics alone in the treatment of an infection are coming to an end. The need to rationalise the use of these drugs is urgent. It takes courage on your part to stop accepting antibiotics as the answer to all infections and to demand a broader approach which includes nutrition, nutritional supplements and natural medicines, as well as comprehensive methods of testing which involve both alternative and conventional medical techniques.

The issue of the side-effects associated with antibiotic use is also of major importance. As the bulk of prescriptions for these drugs are for childhood infections, the damage they are doing to young children concerns me greatly. I consider it important enough to write a separate book on this subject as a body of interesting information is beginning to appear in the medical literature. This book will spell out the reality of using antibiotics and the negative effects they can have on the human body.

Meanwhile, please be aware that in many cases, especially with childhood infections, antibiotics are being prescribed inappropriately. According to the Irish government's Medical Services Annual Report, the most commonly prescribed drug in Ireland for the last three years has been amoxycillin, an antibiotic. Approximately £3 million is spent by the government every year on this drug alone. Other antibiotics also rank highly on the list of most commonly prescribed drugs in Ireland. Isn't it time we asked why such drugs rank top of the list? While I do not have figures for private sector medicine, I would guess that antibiotics also rank highly in this top ten list.

In earlier chapters, I explained the problem of resistance to antibiotics and the urgent need to take action. I also showed that many infections, especially childhood infections, should not be treated with antibiotics. The majority of infections respond very well to natural medicines. I will discuss some of these natural medicines and the ways in which they work in the next few chapters. Let's begin by looking at herbal medicine.

6   *Herbal Medicine*

'The mother of all medicine'

Herbal medicine is the oldest and most tried and tested form of medicine. In a sense it is degrading to refer to it as an 'alternative', since it forms the basis of all medicine—conventional drugs, homeopathic medicine, traditional Chinese medicines, etc. It is the original medicine, the mother of all remedies used today. Herbal medicine has been used by all cultures for centuries and is still the main form of medical treatment among 80% of the world's population. It is sad to hear some doctors describing herbal medicine as quackery since many of today's drugs (e.g. quinine, reserpine, ephedrine, ipecac) come directly from plants, while most synthetic drugs are based on chemicals extracted from herbs. Why has the medical profession not embraced herbal medicines in the same way it has synthetically-produced drugs? I believe the answer has to do with money and power, although teaching methods in medical schools are also a factor.

First of all, there is no big money in herbs. Herbal medicines cannot be patented so there is no incentive to produce them on a large scale. Drugs, regardless of whether they are produced synthetically or isolated from herbal extracts, can be patented, bottled and sold for incredible sums of money. This is what pharmaceutical companies do. This is why they are so wealthy and capable of financing so many medical projects.

The way in which doctors are educated at medical school is another reason why herbal medicine has not been embraced by the medical profession. Medical education is not holistic. It makes no attempt to deal with people on anything other than a physical level. The main form of treatment, even when dealing with sensitive emotional issues, is pharmaceutical drugs. No attempt is made to educate doctors in issues as fundamental as nutrition. You only have to look at the food served in hospital canteens and coffee shops to see the incredible lack of awareness among doctors in this regard—ironically it is often their job to treat people with nutritional imbalances.

Herbal medicine and nutrition must form the cornerstone of medical therapeutics if people are to be *healed* as distinct from *treated*. At present, the only form of therapeutics taught to medical students in university is pharmacology—the study and use of chemical drugs. The medical profession must choose between money and power on the one hand and the good of humanity on the other. When next you see negative reports in the media about herbal medicine, remember that this is the most important form of medicine for the majority of people on the planet, especially those who cannot afford expensive drugs.

The regard which the modern medical establishment holds for herbal medicine is clearly reflected in the attitude of the National Cancer Institute in the U.S. On the one hand, they issue statements confirming that up to 60% of cancers in humans can be prevented by better nutrition and a less stressful lifestyle. This is quite an admission by a body of scientists and doctors who are provided with large sums of money to find *cures* for these cancers. The very same body of people spend approximately 1% of their budget on nutritional research. If this is not revealing enough, the same institute spends vast amounts of money isolating chemicals from herbs which grow in the Amazon River basin of South America. Using the herbs themselves would not produce sufficient profits and that, after all, is what is necessary!

In Chapter 8, which deals with nutrition, I state that

manufacturers of processed foods are interested in profits, not in your health. Unfortunately, it appears that the same can be said of modern medicine and pharmaceutics. Huge sums of money are being spent on isolating chemicals from herbs which are known to have anti-cancer properties. These chemicals are then mass produced, packaged and sold for enormous profits. Using the natural herb is safer and healthier. If the natural herb is used alongside nutritional medicine and changes in lifestyle, the patient can participate in his/her own care and use fewer toxic substances to heal his/her body. The Gerson diet[5], for example, has a higher success rate than chemotherapy, surgery or radiation in the treatment of cancer.

Herbs — part of Nature's energy cycle

All life on this planet depends on the sun. The sun provides us with light and heat energy. Plants use light energy to make food in an amazing process called photosynthesis. This process converts energy into matter (food). In addition to being vital for our survival, photosynthesis beautifully exemplifies one of Albert Einstein's theories—that energy and matter are the same thing, and that one can be converted into the other.

While photosynthesis shows how energy can be converted into matter, there is another remarkable process which can convert matter (food) back into energy. This process is called respiration. When we eat the food in a plant, it is broken down into smaller units (digested) and eventually ends up being used in respiration to provide energy for the body. Many forms of alternative medicine use both matter (a herb, for example) and energy (e.g. homeopathic medicine) to heal people. Scientists who have difficulty in understanding how energy-based medicine such as homeopathy and acupuncture work need only revise basic biology and physics.

---

[5] The Gerson diet utilises the juices of organically-grown fruits and vegetables to help patients overcome cancer. It has achieved great recognition, particularly in the U.S.

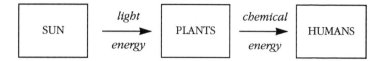

Figure 6.1

Figure 6.1 illustrates an important point—when you use herbs or plants for healing you are part of an energy transfer and, therefore, part of Nature. This energy is universal (from the sun in this example) and flows through Nature to you. By using the herb, you are actually part of something much greater—you are linked into something happening millions of miles from earth. This is why natural medicines are so wonderful to use—they work at different levels within you, not just the physical.

Herbal medicines and synthetic drugs: a comparison

In 1874, sodium salicylate (synthetic aspirin) was synthesised chemically in a laboratory for the first time. This led to a surge in the use of synthetic medicines and a decline in the use of herbs. We assumed that all our medicines could be produced in laboratories and that Nature would become redundant. Gradually, however, this assumption has been dispelled. The thalidomide disaster in the 1950s was a major warning sign of the dangers of using synthetically-produced medicines. In the 1980s, Opren—an anti-inflammatory drug used to treat arthritis—killed a number of patients suffering from that condition. In June 1986, all children's medicine containing aspirin had to be taken off the market because a number of children had died from brain and liver damage (Reye's Syndrome). The problem of side-effects has weakened considerably the arguments in favour of using synthetic drugs. Today, most people are justifiably concerned about the use of conventional medicines.

Not all aspects of chemical analysis and laboratory research are negative, though. In fact, the scientific knowledge we have gained has been of considerable value. It has, for example, proven beyond doubt the claims made by ancient healers about certain plants. The shamans (traditional doctors) of the North American Indians have claimed that plants such as *Echinacea purpurea* and *Baptisia tinctoria* can be used to treat infections. Scientific researchers have isolated particular chemicals (called glycoproteins and polysaccharides) from these herbs and found that they stimulate the immune system as well as damaging invading bacteria. Hence, modern techniques have substantiated what 'primitive' healers have been saying for some time—that these herbs are effective in the treatment of infections. These two herbs are discussed later in this chapter.

Scientists have also analysed a herb called Meadowsweet (*Filipendula ulmaria*) and found that it contains a natural aspirin—it can therefore be used as a pain-killer. The beauty of this analysis is that it has also shown that Meadowsweet contains tannin and mucilage, both of which act to protect the lining of the stomach. Hence, Meadowsweet does not produce the side-effects seen when synthetic aspirin is used. Remedies based on chemicals will never compare with the beauty and intelligence of natural medicines. Daniel Mowrey's excellent book, *The Scientific Validation of Herbal Medicine*, should convince even the most sceptical reader of the validity of herbal medicine.

Table 6.1 below briefly compares conventional and herbal medicine.

Table 6.1 Conventional drugs v herbal medicines

Conventional Drugs	Herbal Medicines
Based on isolated chemicals	Based on the whole plant
Many now made synthetically	All are natural
Not part of the natural energy cycle and so are deficient in energy	All are energy-rich as they use the sun's energy

Use unnaturally high concentrations of a chemical which can disturb a natural system like the body, causing side-effects	Use natural concentrations and so are much safer for for the body
Are more dramatic in their action as they enter the bloodstream rapidly	Are slower to work
Lower the vitality of the body and increase the work of elimination	Enhance the vitality of the body by providing minerals and vitamins

Herbal medicine and intuition

If a dog has eaten meat that has gone off, it will take some Couchgrass (*Agropyron repens*) to make itself vomit. It knows instinctively which plant to eat to treat itself. Similarly, primitive people know which plants to use to cure different ailments. Our ancestors had a similar wealth of knowledge which was handed down from generation to generation. This intuitive knowledge must be respected. Science has tried to diminish its importance and to substitute analysis for intuition. We know instinctively what our bodies need to stay healthy. Trusting these instincts is not so easy, however. As children we were not encouraged to be trusting, so we find this very difficult as adults.

Natural medicine is more an art than a science. Doctors, therapists and healers must have a well-developed sense of intuition to work in this area. The reverse is true of conventional medicine which has allowed itself to become very scientific. A marriage of the two can result in a harmony between art and science, between intuitive ability and scientific skills.

Let's take a look at particular herbs which have been used for centuries to treat infectious diseases. I shall begin by discussing one of the most famous herbs of all, Echinacea.

Echinacea purpurea — the immune herb

Echinacea is famous for its ability to fight infection and to boost the immune system. It is one of the most commonly prescribed herbs in the world, particularly in the U.S. and Germany, although it is not as well known in other parts of Europe. This is probably because Echinacea is indigenous to North America, where it has been used for centuries by the native North Americans in the treatment of infections, skin wounds and snake bites. A German doctor, Dr Meyer, learned about it from the Pawnee tribe and produced a medicine called 'Meyer's Blood Purifier'. By the turn of the century, many doctors were using Echinacea and by 1907 it had become the most popular herb in medical practice. As a result of Dr Meyer's influence, the herb became popular in Germany and today more than 250 medical products in Germany contain Echinacea.

HOW DOES ECHINACEA WORK?

Echinacea stimulates the white blood cells, which help to fight infections in the body. Recent research has shown that it enhances the activity of a particular type of white blood cell —macrophages. In December 1984, the medical journal *Infection and Immunity* reported that a particular ingredient of Echinacea significantly increased the killing effect of macrophages on tumour cells.

WHAT IS ECHINACEA USED FOR?

Because Echinacea can assist in the body's defences, it helps to control viral, bacterial and fungal infections. It is also used for skin wounds and can even be used to treat eczema.

Table 6.2 Uses of Echinacea

Infections	Wounds	Others
colds and 'flu	burns	allergies
sinusitis	skin ulcers	eczema
sore throats	bites and stings	low white blood
ear infections		cell count
staphylococcal infections		
urinary tract infections		

Echinacea is best taken as a liquid extract or tincture. In liquid form, it is more easily absorbed into the bloodstream and as a medicine it will have a longer shelf-life. I find that I get much better results with it as an alcohol extract than in dry (capsule or tablet) form.

Of great importance with any herb are its quality and freshness. I generally use the root of the plant *Echinacea purpurea*. In certain cases I will combine it with *Echinacea angustifolia*, as there is now evidence to suggest that the two are best used together to treat certain conditions. Echinacea in capsule or tablet form is used mainly by patients who cannot tolerate the taste of the liquid extract, but this is quite rare.

Occasionally I use Echinacea alone but more often I combine it with other herbs. For example, in the treatment of sinusitis I combine it with Golden Seal or Marshmallow. For certain respiratory tract infections, it is best combined with Wild Indigo. For immune enhancement, I combine it with Astralagus/Wild Indigo/Myrrh and for lymphatic drainage, I combine it with Cleavers or Poke Root.

Is Echinacea safe to use?

Echinacea is generally recognised as being one of the safest herbs. Many tests have shown it to be non-toxic and in the last five years, I myself have seen no side-effects at all.

Summary

Echinacea is one of the most important natural remedies for treating both acute and recurrent infections. It is effective against a wide range of microbes, including many viruses, bacteria and fungi. It can be used internally to treat infections anywhere in the body and can also be used for external conditions as an ointment or salve.

It is described as the herb that will convince even the most sceptical of doctors and, as such, has done much to convert many conventional doctors to natural medicine.

Wild Indigo (*Baptisia tinctoria*)

This is another North American plant which has been used by the indigenous peoples for centuries. The Creek Indians, for example, used to give an extract of the root to children showing signs of an infection, to help them fight it. Wild Indigo was also used by other tribes, mainly for infections but also to treat wounds and bruises.

Wild Indigo is virtually unknown as a medicinal herb in Europe, although it has been used in German homeopathic medicine since the mid-1800s. Like *Echinacea purpurea*, the active constituents of Wild Indigo are in the roots. The chemicals which stimulate the immune system consist of glycoproteins and to a lesser extent polysaccharides—the chemical structures of these have now been determined through scientific research.

How does Wild Indigo work?

Wild Indigo has an antibiotic-like effect on a wide range of microbes, including many bacteria and fungi. As such it has a killing effect on the microbe, preventing it from multiplying in the body. It also has an immune-enhancing effect and some of the chemicals in Wild Indigo have a strong anti-catarrhal effect. It is interesting to note that many of the anti-infective herbs simultaneously stimulate one's immunity. This is the beauty of using natural remedies.

Taking Wild Indigo orally, as a tincture or alcoholic extract, can lead to a 30% increase in the number of white blood cells—they fight infection—within two to three hours of taking the substance. This data is supported by further research from other studies. Using a homeopathic preparation of the herb produces a similar result.

More recent research on Wild Indigo glycoproteins appears to indicate that the lymphocytes (a particular type of white blood cell) are the white cells most activated by the plant extract.

What is Wild Indigo used for?

Because of its antibiotic and anti-catarrhal effects, Wild

Indigo is most useful for infections of the respiratory tract. It is effective in the treatment of various acute and chronic infections—of the sinuses (sinusitis), the lining of the nose (rhinitis), the back of the throat (tonsillitis, pharyngitis) and the lower respiratory tract (laryngitis, tracheitis and bronchitis).

I have found it especially beneficial in the treatment of infections associated with the production of large amounts of catarrh in the ear, nose, throat and sinuses (upper respiratory tract). I have also used it as a mouthwash to heal mouth ulcers and to treat gingivitis.

Like Echinacea, Wild Indigo can also be used externally. It can be applied, as an ointment or salve, to treat skin infections, wounds, and sore nipples in mothers who are breast-feeding.

Table 6.3 Uses of Wild Indigo

Respiratory tract infections
 sinusitis
 tonsillitis
 rhinitis
 bronchitis

Skin infections
 wounds
 infected eczema
 sore nipples

Mouthwash for mouth infections

Immune booster

How do you take Wild Indigo?

For maximum benefit, Wild Indigo is best used as a tincture or liquid extract, like Echinacea. It can, however, be used as a powder or in capsule/tablet form. The roots of this herb are usually dug up in the autumn, cleaned and dried and then chewed or ground up into a powder. It is also used in this form to make a liquid extract which can be taken internally.

The freshness of the herb is an important consideration. A

liquid extract will have a much longer shelf-life, approximately one to two years, whereas the capsules or tablets have a much shorter period of usefulness. If using the latter, check the expiry date.

For the treatment of infections, I often combine Wild Indigo with Echinacea or Myrrh.

IS WILD INDIGO SAFE TO USE?
Like Echinacea, Wild Indigo has a wonderful safety record. It can be used with confidence for the above-mentioned infections in both adults and children, even very young children, at the correct dosage. Excessively high doses may be less safe.

SUMMARY
Wild Indigo has antibiotic and immune-stimulating effects as well as anti-catarrhal properties. It is used to treat catarrhal infections of the respiratory tract, skin and mouth infections. It is best taken as a liquid extract. It is very safe to use in adults and children although very high doses may be less safe.

Usnea barbata — the herbal antibiotic
Usnea barbata is a lichen which grows from trees in the forests and orchards of Northern Europe. Because it hangs in long, grey strands from the branches of trees such as pine, oak, fir and apple, it is often called 'Old Man's Beard' or larch moss.

Lichens are not really plants. They are two plant-like structures, a fungus and an alga, living together. The two become so interwoven that they act like a single plant. Some lichens are bright yellow or red and are used to make the dye for Scottish and Irish tweeds.

HOW DOES USNEA WORK?
Usnea barbata is a very effective antibiotic and truly deserves to be called 'the herbal antibiotic'. It produces a substance called usnic acid which has proven to be more powerful than penicillin against certain bacteria. Its action is similar to

penicillin in that it disrupts or destroys bacterial and fungal cells. So, we can say that Usnea has a penicillin-like action.

What is Usnea used for?

Research has shown that Usnea is most effective against certain bacteria—*Staphylococcus spp.*, *Streptococcus spp.* and *Mycobacterium tuberculosis* (which causes TB). In some cases, it is more effective than penicillin. Usnea has also been shown to be superior to conventional drugs, such as metronidazole (Flagyl), in the treatment of *Trichomonas* infections of the vagina and cervix.

Because of its very strong antibiotic effect, it is particularly useful in the treatment of bacterial or fungal infections, such as bacterial sinusitis/tonsillitis and bacterial pneumonia, as well as bacterial skin infections, such as Staphylococcal boils and abscesses, fungal ringworm and athlete's foot. It is interesting to note that many of the anti-fungal creams on the market today have Usnea as a constituent.

Usnea is *not* effective in the treatment of urinary tract infections as these are caused by a different type of bacteria, usually *E. coli.*

How do you take Usnea?

Usnea is best used as a tincture. Take a dropful of the tincture (ten drops) in a little water, two to three times daily, for acute bacterial infections. A dropful in a little water can be used as a gargle for sore throats, especially a streptococcal throat. For a sinus infection a dropful in a little water can be instilled into the nasal passages several times a day. A dropful in water can also be used as a douche, to treat vaginal infections.

Is Usnea safe to use?

Yes, but it is best used under medical supervision as it can cause gastro-intestinal upsets in some people. Hence, it is sometimes best to start with a lower dose and gradually work up to the recommended dose over a few days.

Because Usnea dissolves poorly in water, an alcohol liquid extract is best. Dilute it before use as it can be irritating to the stomach if swallowed undiluted.

At very high doses, Usnea can be toxic. If used as an alcohol extract, there is no cause for concern, as it is absorbed quite slowly. I always advise patients never to use it without medical supervision.

SUMMARY
Usnea barbata is a lichen found hanging from trees. It is often called 'Old Man's Beard' or larch moss. Its main constituent is usnic acid, a very effective antibiotic. It is used to treat certain bacterial infections, fungal infections and vaginal infections. Usnea is quite safe but it is best used under medical supervision.

Usnea can, in some cases, be more effective than an antibiotic such as penicillin.

Myrrh (*Commiphora molmol*)

Myrrh comes from a completely different part of the world—the 'gold, frankincense and myrrh' part. This plant grows as a bush in the arid regions of Arabia, the Middle East and northeast Africa. The people of this region have been collecting the gum resin from this plant for centuries and have used it to treat a range of infections. The gum is often referred to as 'gugal gum' and the plant is sometimes called 'Guggulu'. The Arabs used it for stomach complaints and for respiratory infections—an arid climate is quite hard on the respiratory system!

How Does Myrrh Work?

Extracts from the plant have been shown to enhance phagocytosis in white blood cells (the killing effect of white blood cells). As such, Myrrh is effective at helping your body to fight a whole range of infections—viral, bacterial and fungal. Like Echinacea, recent research has indicated that it also has a direct anti-microbial effect.

What is Myrrh Used For?

Of the herbs discussed so far, Myrrh is the strongest agent for treating skin infections.

Table 6.4 Uses of Myrrh

Upper respiratory tract infections
  sinusitis

Lower respiratory tract infections
  bronchitis

Streptococcal infections
  sore throats

Staphylococcal infections
  boils
  abscesses

Viral infections
  'flu
  common cold
  Herpes simplex

HOW DO YOU TAKE MYRRH?
Because the resin does not dissolve well in water, it is best used as an alcohol extract (tincture). The recommended dosage is 2–4 ml of this tincture taken three times daily. It is best used in combination with other herbs and is often combined with Wild Indigo for respiratory tract infections, or with Echinacea for other infections.

IS MYRRH SAFE TO USE?
Myrrh is very safe. No toxic effects or side-effects have been recorded.

SUMMARY
Myrrh originates from Arabia and north-east Africa. It has a direct anti-microbial effect as well as enhancing the killing action of white blood cells. The Arabs used it mainly for respiratory infections but it can be used for a wide range of infections. The gum resin dissolves poorly in water, so the alcohol extract is the best form to use. Combine it with Wild Indigo for respiratory infections and with Echinacea for other infections.

Other medicinal herbs

So far we have looked at four herbs that are often used to treat infections. There are a host of others that are used less commonly, including Sage, Thyme, Marigold, Wormwood and Garlic. Thuja is another herb that I shall discuss separately. It has well established anti-viral properties.

Sage (Salvia officinalis) and Thyme (Thymus vulgaris)

Both Sage and Thyme are strongly antiseptic and can be used as effective gargles for sore throats, including bacterial (streptococcal) tonsillitis. They can be taken internally for both upper and lower respiratory tract infections and can be used externally for skin infections.

Sage is an excellent remedy for inflammatory conditions of the mouth and throat. It can be used as a mouthwash for gingivitis (inflamed gums) and for stomatitis (inflammation of the lining of the mouth). It is an excellent remedy for mouth ulcers (aphthous ulcers).

Thyme is an excellent cough remedy. If the cough is associated with the production of phlegm (a wet cough), this herb aids the removal of phlegm from the body. If the cough is dry and irritating, it will have a soothing effect. Thyme is one of the best antiseptic substances available, which makes it valuable in the treatment of infections.

Marigold (Calendula officinalis)

Marigold has marked anti-fungal properties and may be used both internally and externally for fungal infections. It is also the herb of choice in the treatment of skin problems—inflammatory skin conditions, skin infections, slow-healing wounds and skin ulcers.

Garlic (Allium sativum)

Garlic is well known for its antibiotic properties. It was used by the ancient Egyptians to treat worm infestations and infections, by the Greeks and Romans for tumours, wounds and generalised infections, and by the Chinese to treat weakness, fatigue, infections and tumours. In 1858, Louis

Pasteur demonstrated the wonderful anti-bacterial properties of garlic. In both World Wars, garlic saved countless thousands of lives by protecting wounds from becoming infected. When no other antiseptic was available, surface wounds were smeared with crushed garlic and then bandaged.

More recent research has shown that garlic juice can slow the growth, or kill, more than sixty species of fungi and more than twenty species of bacteria, including some of the most virulent. Interestingly, garlic is currently attracting a lot of attention from the medical profession for its ability to lower blood cholesterol as well as for its anti-cancer properties.

The oil in garlic contains the active substance responsible for its antibiotic/anti-microbial properties. This oil contains a sulphur compound called allicin which kills bacteria and fungi. When eaten, the oil enters the digestive system and is absorbed into the bloodstream. It is excreted via the lungs, hence the strong sulphur-type odour of the breath. Because of this, garlic is best used for infections of the digestive and respiratory tracts.

WORMWOOD (*ARTEMISIA ABSINTHUM*)
As the name suggests, Wormwood is a good remedy for worm infestation, especially roundworms. Because it has such a bitter taste, it is best to take it in tablet form.

SUMMARY
There are a number of plants which have strong antibiotic and immune-strengthening properties. Used correctly, these herbs form the basis for all natural antibiotics. It is fascinating to discover that many of the helpful chemicals in these plants are of little benefit to the plant itself. Many of these chemicals have been produced by the plants to assist the rest of Nature. The beauty and wisdom of the natural world is astonishing!

Thuja occidentalis
This herb is also known as the Tree of Life (*Arbor vitae*). A woody plant, belonging to the Cypress family, it is native to

the north-eastern part of North America. It is cultivated in Europe as a garden plant, particularly as hedging, so you may already be familiar with it.

Thuja was imported to Europe during the sixteenth century and became well known medicinally as a homeopathic preparation. In its country of origin, it was used mainly as a herbal preparation. When taken internally in high dosages, or in lower dosages over a long period of time, herbal preparations of Thuja were found to cause severe side-effects. These do not occur when Thuja is applied externally to the skin or when it is used as a homeopathic preparation. Hence it is safe to use Thuja as a homeopathic preparation but *not* as a herbal extract. The latter is safe to use on skin lesions only.

The positive influence of Thuja applied topically to skin conditions, warts and genital warts has been described in numerous articles. As far back as 1838, a Dr Warnatz reported a patient with exceedingly refractory warts (i.e. unresponsive to treatment) on the penis and scrotum which were healed with Thuja.

Good results have been reported by numerous researchers since then. Most of the research relating to Thuja centres on the treatment of skin warts and the use of Thuja as an external application, rather than as an internal medicine. In 1949, Halter described the treatment of warts using Thuja internally, without any external application at all. It is now believed that Thuja has an inhibitory action on viruses. It can therefore be taken internally for a whole range of viral diseases of the respiratory tract, digestive tract and the skin in particular.

How does Thuja work?
Thuja has been investigated mostly as an anti-viral substance. Unequivocal evidence of its strong anti-viral properties was presented by Khurana (1971), who investigated the effects of this herb on a host of different viruses. Others have confirmed this anti-viral effect, although the active chemicals have not yet been identified. According to some researchers, Thuja possesses anti-bacterial properties as well, so it may be

useful in the treatment of infected surface wounds and burns.

Despite centuries of use, in folk medicine and homeopathy, little scientific research has been done on Thuja compared to that done on other herbs like Echinacea, for example.

WHAT IS THUJA USED FOR?

Thuja is used mainly for viral infections. If you have a cold, 'flu, viral sore throat, viral laryngitis or viral bronchitis, then it should be taken internally as a homeopathic preparation.

For viral skin infections such as warts and genital warts, it can be applied directly to the wart. When applied directly to the skin, it can be used as a herbal extract. The herb also has a marked anti-fungal effect and so is useful for external fungal infections like ringworm.

Another effect which has been well documented in the scientific literature is the ability of Thuja to prevent a common tropical disease called bilharzia. This is caused by a worm, the larvae of which can penetrate human skin when in contact with fresh water. When applied to the skin, Thuja has been shown to prevent the larva from penetrating the skin.

Thuja has also been reported to counteract the ill effects of smallpox vaccination.

HOW DO YOU TAKE THUJA?

Thuja is best taken internally as homeopathic drops or applied externally in the form of a liquid herbal extract. It can also be taken internally as a herbal extract, primarily to treat viral infections of the respiratory tract, but this should only be *done under medical supervision.*

IS THUJA SAFE TO USE?

Thuja is one herb which is best administered by a doctor or qualified herbalist, especially if it is being taken as an oral medicine. Research has shown that if a cold water/alcohol extraction method is used in preparing the herbal medicine, the side-effects are absent, making it much safer to take orally.

SUMMARY

Thuja has been used in American folk medicine for centuries, and in Europe as a homeopathic preparation since the early 1800s. Its main benefit appears to be its ability to treat all viral infections. Hence, it is used for bronchitis, laryngitis and sore throats of viral origin. It can be applied externally to treat skin warts and genital warts, and fungal infections such as ringworm.

It is safe to use as homeopathic drops but *requires medical supervision* if used internally as a herbal extract.

Esberitox — an exciting new herbal immune stimulant

Esberitox is a relatively new herbal medicine containing extracts from Echinacea, Wild Indigo and Thuja. Now on the market in Europe, it is produced in the form of drops and tablets.

I was excited about this product when I first heard of it, as I was relieved to find that someone somewhere was thinking along lines similar to myself. During the last five years I have seen a particular need for Echinacea and Wild Indigo among my patients, so it is good to be able to use a product which combines the immune-enhancing properties of these with a third herb, Thuja, which has become well known for its anti-viral properties.

WHAT DOES ESBERITOX CONTAIN?

Esberitox contains extracts from three different herbs—Echinacea, Wild Indigo and Thuja. All of these herbs have an immune-stimulating effect.

HOW DOES ESBERITOX WORK?

The active chemicals in Esberitox (glycoproteins and polysaccharides) have the ability to attach themselves to the surface of certain cells in the immune system (macrophages). These chemicals then activate the immune system, protecting against infection and shortening the duration of an existing infection. The manufacturers of Esberitox recommend its use in conjunction with an antibiotic, especially for severe bacterial infections. I would endorse this, but as I said earlier, most infections—especially respiratory infections in children—are viral and so, these herbal substances alone would be sufficient.

Esberitox can be used for a variety of ailments as outlined in the table below.

Table 6.5 Uses of Esberitox

Acute and chronic respiratory tract infections
Severe bacterial infections (in conjunction with an antibiotic)
   streptococcal sore throat
   otitis media (middle ear infection)
Bacterial skin infections
   boils
   abscesses
   impetigo
To reduce susceptibility to infection (due to lowered
   resistance)
*To enhance the white blood cell count following anti-cancer
   treatment* (with radiotherapy and/or chemotherapy)

ARE THERE SIDE-EFFECTS?
No side-effects have been recorded with the oral use of Esberitox. If it is administered intravenously, which is rare, a short-term reaction may occur in some cases. This is regarded as a desired or positive reaction in natural medicine, so it is not viewed as a side-effect in the usual sense of the word, which implies a negative or harmful effect. However, as Esberitox contains Thuja which can stimulate the uterus wall to contract, this product is best avoided during pregnancy.

SUMMARY
Esberitox has an important role to play in bacterial and viral infections. It not only has immune-stimulating properties, it

has anti-viral and anti-bacterial properties also. It is very useful for cancer patients who have undergone chemotherapy or radiotherapy and is also important in treating patients with a lowered resistance.

Case History 6

Jennifer — Glandular fever

Thirteen-year-old Jennifer had been diagnosed as having glandular fever by her family doctor. This is a viral illness that causes a fever and enlarged, tender lymph glands in the early stages. It may also cause liver and spleen enlargement. Glandular fever is a severe illness and it can take months for a patient to completely recover. Later, it can go on to cause chronic fatigue. Jennifer's blood tests showed that the virus was still active in her body.

Initially, I prescribed two measures to treat Jennifer—an immune booster and high-dose vitamin C (the vitamin C needs of the body increase considerably during an infection). This resulted in a marked improvement in her symptoms and she was able to return to school. Within six weeks, her blood tests returned to normal, but she still complained of discomfort in the upper right quadrant of the abdomen. On examination, her liver was still enlarged and tender. I gave her Milk Thistle (*Silybum marianum*), a wonderful herb at assisting liver function. Two months later Jennifer was fully recovered.

Immunol — a powerful immune booster

Immunol is another exciting product that I have recently started to use. It differs from Esberitox in that it has a stronger effect on the immune system. I consider it more exciting because the herbs used in this product are grown organically and are 'energy enriched'. Not only do the manufacturers of this product have a great understanding of the physical constituents of herbs, they also understand the energy properties of plants. For example, the plants used in Immunol are harvested at a particular time of the month and the extracts are exposed to the rising Sun in the morning and to the setting Sun in the evening for the following two weeks, in order to energise them. Many herbal and homeopathic medicine producers are aware that these two times of the day have a high energy level but few actually utilise this fact in the production of medicines. It is wonderful to see this awareness finally being used to make better medicines for all of us.

Immunol was the immune booster I used to treat Jennifer, the young girl discussed in Case History 6. I have since used it on a number of my patients and can testify that it is indeed an amazing medicine.

WHAT DOES IMMUNOL CONTAIN?

Immunol contains extracts from *Echinacea purpurea*, *Echinacea angustifolia*, *Baptisia tinctoria* and *Thuja occidentalis*, all of which are subjected to the special energy-enriching process described above. Research suggests that the two species of Echinacea (*Echinacea purpurea* and *Echinacea angustifolia)* have a more powerful effect on the immune system when combined together as they appear to be synergistic (i.e. one boosts the effects of the other). This makes Immunol a rather unique product as I know of no other immune stimulant that contains both herbal extracts. In addition, Immunol contains *Baptisia tinctoria* and *Thuja occidentalis* the benefits of which have already been discussed.

WHAT IS IMMUNOL USED FOR?

Immunol is particularly useful in the treatment of allergies and recurrent infections. Generally speaking though, it has a wide range of applications as Table 6.6 shows.

Table 6.6 Uses of Immunol

To treat an existing bacterial, viral or fungal infection
To prevent the recurrence of an infection
To assist patients who suffer from allergies (e.g. asthma, eczema, hayfever and sinusitis)

To assist with convalescence from a serious illness

To protect the immune system during periods of stress

To boost the immune system during anti-cancer treatment
(radiotherapy or chemotherapy)

ARE THERE SIDE EFFECTS?
No side effects have been recorded with the use of Immunol whether taken as a liquid or in tablet form. However, because Immunol contains the herb Thuja the cautionary note mentioned for Esberitox also applies here—avoid Immunol during pregnancy as it can cause uterine contractions.

SUMMARY
Because the herbal constituents of Immunol are grown organically and are energised in a special way, this product is unique in its ability to boost the body's defences. Immunol is also unique because it contains two species of the herb Echinacea, which are known to act in a synergistic manner.

It comes in the form of tablets or drops and is very safe to use in both adults and children. It should not be used during pregnancy, though, as it can cause the womb to contract. While it is especially useful for people with allergies and for those who suffer from recurrent infections, it actually has a wide range of applications. It is a product I wholly approve of as I support organic methods of cultivation and I support the thought and energy that goes into its production.

Summary

When I was at medical school I learned ways to *suppress* the immune system with drugs such as steroids, azathioprine and cyclosporin which are used in transplant patients and in the treatment of certain auto-immune diseases. I did not learn how to *enhance* one's immunity. It was only years later I discovered that there are in fact ways to boost one's immunity.

It is encouraging to see herbs such as Echinacea, Wild Indigo and Thuja being more commonly used by patients to

77

protect themselves and their families. Encourage your family doctor to learn more about these herbs so that he/she may prescribe them for you too. Because of the high level of safety associated with Echinacea and Wild Indigo, you may use them without a prescription. If in doubt, consult a medical herbalist, pharmacist or doctor trained in natural medicine.

7

Homeopathic
Medicine

'Small is beautiful'

Unlike Germany and the U.S., Ireland does not have a tradition in homeopathy. As a consequence, this form of medicine is not commonly understood by people in Ireland. It is still in its infancy here, but in Britain there are four homeopathic hospitals, a training school for doctors (at the Royal London Homeopathic Hospital), and treatment is available under the National Health Service. Many British doctors also do training courses in homeopathy and natural medicine in Germany, Austria and France. In these countries, a large percentage of doctors practise homeopathy, either as part of a general practice or full-time like myself.

For the most part, homeopathic medicines are derived from herbs. A few are also derived from minerals such as sulphur and phosphorus. Minute doses of these are used to stimulate the healing powers of the body in a very specific way. For example, if you have a cough a homeopath will use a remedy to stimulate the cough, explaining that the cough is the body's way of expelling an irritant (a virus, inhaled dust, smoke) out of the airway. In other words, homeopathic medicines stimulate the body to heal itself. Echinacea and Wild Indigo, herbs you have already read about, are often used in homeopathic form to stimulate the body's defences in cases of infection.

Simply explained, homeopathic medicines enhance your own natural healing powers. They are very safe, even in new-born babies, as they have *no side-effects*. They come in many different forms, including tablets, drops, ampoules, suppositories and nasal sprays, much like conventional medicines.

Simple and complex homeopathy
There are two different forms of homeopathy currently being practised in Europe. The classical or more traditional form is called simple homeopathy. This type of homeopathy is based on a single remedy being used at any one time. A simple homeopath will select a remedy on the basis of a detailed history from the patient—he/she must try to match the patient's symptoms with a particular remedy.

The newer approach is called complex homeopathy and involves the use of more than one remedy at a time. The majority of homeopathic doctors in Europe today practise complex homeopathy primarily because it works more rapidly.

In the table below you can see examples of one simple and two complex homeopathic remedies. The simple remedy contains one substance, in one strength or potency —Echinacea at a strength of 10× in this case (7.1a). A complex remedy can contain a number of different substances (7.1c) or different strengths of the same substance (7.1b).

Table 7.1 Simple v complex homeopathic remedies

| Simple | Complex | |
7.1(a)	7.1(b)	7.1(c)
Echinacea 10×	Echinacea 10×	Echinacea 10×
	Echinacea 30×	Baptisia 10×
	Echinacea 100×	Bryonia 30×

Complex homeopathic remedies
I prescribe a number of complex homeopathic remedies in my practice. For adults and children with acute infections, I

often prescribe a remedy called Toxiloges. For children with recurrent infections, I prescribe Echinacea compositum. These two products are produced in Germany and are rather similar in action.

Toxiloges is useful in treating both bacterial and viral infections. It is especially useful as a prophylactic in people who are prone to recurrent infections. It can also be used to shorten the recovery period after a serious infection.

Table 7.2 outlines some of the situations in which Toxiloges is used.

Table 7.2 Uses for Toxiloges

Infectious disease
    colds and chills
    bronchitis
    tonsillitis
    infectious childhood disease—mumps, measles
    local infections—boils, abscesses

Prophylactic—to prevent infection

To shorten convalescence

Toxiloges contains a number of homeopathic substances, some of which are derived from herbs (you will probably recognise the names of some of these herbs).
- Echinacea—an immune booster
- Wild Indigo—the remedy of choice in catarrhal infections and localised infections like sinusitis
- Bryonia—for catarrhal symptoms of mucosa
- Eupatorium—also anti-catarrhal
- Ipecacuanha—expectorant and so useful if treating a cough
- Other constituents

Toxiloges contains the anti-infective and immune-enhancing substances, Echinacea and Wild Indigo. It also contains Bryonia and Eupatorium, both of which have an anti-catarrhal action on the mucosa which lines the respiratory tract.

The second complex remedy that I use frequently is called Echinacea compositum, a medicine familiar to a number of my patients. Like Toxiloges, it has a broad spectrum of action.

Echinacea compositum contains the same substances as Toxiloges, but has the added benefit of the following ingredients.

- Lachesis (snake venom)—an excellent remedy for septic illness
- Thuja (Tree of Life)—anti-viral; important where an infection has been treated with antibiotics
- Poke Root (*Phytolacca americana*)—to drain enlarged lymph glands
- Nosodes or vaccines against the bacteria *Streptococcus spp.* and *Staphylococcus spp.*
- Also contains an anti-flu nosode (vaccine)

Echinacea compositum contains Lachesis, Thuja and Poke Root. These are combined with Cleavers (*Galium aparine*), which is excellent at clearing the lymph glands of infection. Echinacea compositum also contains nosodes or vaccines to treat streptococcal, staphylococcal and influenza-type infections. It is a marvellous substance and one which is essential for any doctor who is serious about treating infections safely. Since the herbal form of Echinacea compositum can have a strong taste in the mouth, we often use the homeopathic form for young children.

ENGYSTOL

Engystol is another complex remedy often used in combination with Echinacea to treat viral infections. It can be used in tablet form or as ampoules. Engystol is effective in the treatment of viral infections such as influenza, the common cold, glandular fever, viral gastro-enteritis, Herpes simplex infections (cold sores), shingles, etc. It is currently under review as an additional treatment for patients with hepatitis and AIDS.

In viral tonsillitis in a child, for example, I would prescribe

Engystol as an anti-viral measure and Echinacea compositum drops and/or ampoules to assist the body's defences. This is a very effective way of overcoming an acute infection quickly. I would then continue the drops for a further seven days to assist the body's recovery. I may use Cleavers in herbal or homeopathic form to drain the lymph glands. The following case history illustrates this approach.

CASE HISTORY 7

Jackie — Tonsillitis

Jackie came to me as the first port of call, not the last, as is the case with so many of my patients. She was suffering from tonsillitis. On examination, the tonsils were inflamed but there was no pus (white dots on the tonsils). She also had enlarged lymph glands and a low-grade temperature. I diagnosed viral tonsillitis and prescribed vitamin C, Echinacea compositum ampoules, and the anti-viral remedy Engystol in ampoule form for five days.

After forty-eight hours of treatment, there was a marked improvement in Jackie's condition. Later I used Cleavers, a herbal medicine, to drain the lymph nodes.

Jackie's case was relatively uncomplicated and it illustrates just how easy it can be to treat an acute infection using natural medicines. Unfortunately, many of my patients problems are much more complicated than this and they sometimes do not respond to such simple measures.

Patients who suffer from recurrent infections, as distinct from a single acute infection, would be treated differently and I shall discuss the management of such patients later.

Children respond so quickly to complex homeopathic medicines that it is a delight to treat them. It is wonderful to be able to prescribe for others medicines I am happy to use on myself. There have been a few occasions over the years when I've had to take these medicines to get over a cold or 'flu. I've found them so useful for myself and my family that we take them wherever we travel. It is particularly rewarding to see my youngest daughter, Marianne, who was so prone to infections earlier in her life, now free of infection and thriving.

ADVERSE EFFECTS OF ANTIBIOTICS

Sometimes it is necessary to treat patients for the adverse effects of antibiotics, like Gerard in Case History 4. There are homeopathic medicines specifically designed to undo the harm that certain antibiotics cause within the body. These homeopathic medicines may even have the same name as the antibiotic, for example, tetracycline. When patients see this name, they get confused and can be anxious that I too am giving them antibiotics. A simple explanation, or showing them a page in my *Materia Medica* (a book containing a list of homeopathic medicines and what they do), alleviates their anxiety.

Table 7.3 lists the more common adverse effects of antibiotic usage that I've seen in my practice.

Table 7.3 Adverse effects of antibiotics

Effects on the respiratory tract
  increased mucus production
  chronic cough
  nasal congestion
  ear-ache
  itchy ears

Effects on the digestive tract
  abdominal pain/discomfort
  sickly feeling in the stomach
  increased flatulence (wind)
  alteration to bacterial flora
  pancreatic damage

Nutritional effects
  a decrease in the level of certain minerals (zinc, calcium, magnesium)
  a decrease in the level of certain vitamins (K, B_2, B_3)

General effects
   tiredness
   altered mood
   impaired immune response

If I see any of these symptoms in a patient, it is a warning to me that antibiotic damage may be present and that a homeopathic 'antidote' may be needed at some stage in the course of treatment.

I remember, in particular, a young man who had been on two separate courses of tetracycline for teenage acne. The first course was for a period of six months, followed eight weeks later by a longer course of twelve months. When a broad-spectrum antibiotic has been used for long periods like this, damage is almost inevitable, especially to the digestive system.

I sent this patient for testing and the results showed both pancreatic damage and alterations to the bacterial flora. Furthermore, testing also indicated the need to use tetracycline in homeopathic form, which I did. This did not solve his acne problem, but it was necessary if this patient was going to show any positive response to medicines specifically for his acne.

Such are the difficulties involved in practising homeopathy. One must first use remedies to boost the patient's level of health (e.g. detoxification remedies) so that when you prescribe a remedy for a particular complaint, it will be much more likely to have a beneficial effect.

Some patients are so toxic that I could spend weeks/months boosting their level of health prior to treating their symptoms. This high level of toxicity may be due to a number of factors—drinking tap water which contains heavy metals and chemicals such as chlorine and fluoride; eating foods with chemical additives; breathing polluted air; using drugs (especially steroids, anti-inflammatory drugs and antibiotics); stressing the body by working long hours; or by taking stimulants such as tea and coffee.

SUMMARY

Complex homeopathy is used to treat acute infections and recurrent infections. It is also used to boost one's defences, to undo the damage that drugs like antibiotics can do to the body and to detoxify (remove toxins from) the body.

Simple homeopathic remedies

With simple homeopathy, a single remedy is used in a single potency or strength. The choice of remedy for a patient depends very much on their symptoms (as Tables 7.4 and 7.5 illustrate). In young children, it is often hard to get an accurate history. Although simple remedies can be slow to work, when they do so, they are very effective.

Table 7.4 Simple homeopathic remedies for tonsillitis

Symptoms	Possible Remedy
where swallowing worsens the sore throat	Lachesis
where swallowing improves the sore throat	Ignatia
where there has been suppression of the symptoms with antibiotics	Thuja
where only the right side of the throat is involved	Lycopodium
where there is oedematous swelling of the tonsils	Apis mellifica

Table 7.5 Simple homeopathic remedies for ear-ache

Symptoms	Possible remedy
where the ear-ache follows a cold or measles and is associated with a yellow discharge; worse at night	Pulsatilla

where the child is irritable and does not want to be held; can be unbearable; worse on bending down	Chamomilla
acute onset of pain; pain is very severe and the child is in a state of anguish; pain may spread into the face or down into the neck	Belladonna

Chamomilla is the remedy of choice for teething in young children. Belladonna is the remedy of choice for scarlet fever. All simple remedies, and some complex remedies, are available from a homeopathic pharmacy. Consult your local homeopathic doctor.

I feel that a broad approach to the patient is necessary, involving diet, lifestyle, mineral and vitamin supplementation (where appropriate). I also feel that a quicker-acting complex remedy, especially in the case of a streptococcal infection of the tonsils, yields much better results. That is why I prefer to use medicines which are specifically anti-infective. These include Echinacea compositum and Toxiloges as well as the herbs you read about earlier.

Homeopathic medicines form the majority of my own prescriptions for patients. I find them extremely effective at treating not just an acute infection, but also in assisting people with chronic infections and recurrent infections. I have mentioned only a few to illustrate how they work. There are, in fact, many other preparations on the market today. Most of them are British, French or German, as most reputable homeopathic medicines in Europe originate in these countries. It is important to use medicines from reputable companies if you want to benefit from this form of medicine.

Karen — recurrent chest infections, tiredness, aches and pains

Karen was only five years old when her mother brought her to me complaining of these symptoms. Examination of the child and a chest X-ray revealed an infection in the lower right lung. I treated this homeopathically and the child responded well.

However, two recurrences in the next two months suggested that there was more going on. I was suspicious that the child's immunity was impaired, so I sent her for electronic testing. This revealed that mercury from the mother's amalgam (dental) fillings had affected the child *in utero* (as a foetus in the mother's womb). A homeopathic detoxification medicine (Metex), specifically designed to remove metals such as mercury from the body, was prescribed. Now, one year later, there have been no recurrences of the chest infection.

This case is interesting in two ways. Firstly, it has taught me to ask about the mother's health during pregnancy, about medications taken, etc. Secondly, I have learned to dig more deeply when looking for the cause of an ailment, especially if a child fails to get better. I have found electronic testing very helpful in this regard, as it can pick up problems that I would have great difficulty detecting using ordinary clinical methods.

Since testing Karen over eighteen months ago, I have discovered a number of other cases of children who were affected by mercury poisoning from their mother's fillings (*in utero*). Mercury is highly toxic and can leak out of fillings into the mouth. Once swallowed, it is absorbed into the bloodstream. In this way, it can cross the placenta and affect the health of the foetus.

The importance of homeopathic vaccination

During the mid-1970s, an epidemic of bacterial meningitis broke out in Brazil. In an attempt to control the spread of the disease, homeopathic doctors inoculated over 18,000 children with a homeopathic nosode (or vaccine) of the bacteria causing meningitis (*Neisseria meningitidis*). This group of children subsequently had a very low incidence of meningitis when compared with other children in the area.

The outcome of this treatment clearly shows the importance of homeopathic medicine and illustrates the need for governments to accept it as a valid form of medicine.

Homeopathic medicine became very popular in Europe and North America because of its success in controlling the cholera epidemics that ravaged these continents during the nineteenth century. Statistics at the time, from hospitals in different parts of Europe, showed that the death rate in homeopathic hospitals was very low compared to that in conventional hospitals. For example, in 1831 in Raab, Hungary, only six out of 154 homeopathically-treated patients died, compared with 59% of those treated conventionally. Elsewhere in Europe, the mortality rate varied between 2% and 20% for those treated homeo-pathically, compared with 50–60% for those treated conventionally. These statistics, which were suppressed by the governments of these countries so as not to discredit conventional medicine, undoubtedly attest to the power of homeopathy.

More recently, Gaucher et al. (1992) found homeopathic medicines to be so effective in treating a cholera epidemic in Peru that they have now begun a large-scale clinical trial. Homeopathic medicines are cheap, effective and easy to use. It makes sense to use them, both in terms of economics and human health.

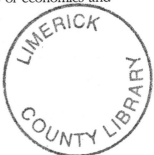

8 Nutritional Medicine

'Healthy food is the best medicine'

Eating and breathing are the two most important things we do every day in order to stay alive. The food with which you nourish your body is of critical importance to your health. Good food—natural foods which Nature intended you to eat —will provide your body with the nutrients essential for good health, particularly an effective immune system. Bad food—unnatural or processed foods—will lead to a steady decline in your health, making you more prone to infections.

After almost twelve years in Africa, I was shocked on my return to Europe to see the kind of foods people were eating here. In Africa, people eat a diet based on natural foods, at least for the most part. They eat a minimum of processed foods as they are too expensive. What grows in the back garden is cheap, but what comes from food processing factories is expensive. In Europe, much of the food that we consume is 'dead' food. It contains too much sugar and much of it is processed.

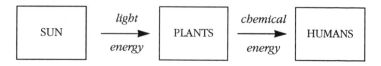

Figure 8.1

All energy on this planet comes from the sun. The sun

provides us with heat and light energy. As Figure 8.1 shows, plants use light energy from the sun to make food in a beautiful process called photosynthesis. During photosynthesis, light energy is converted to chemical energy. This energy is passed along to us when we eat the plant. Hence, we refer to natural foods as being energy-rich. Put simply, the sun's energy ends up in your body, keeping it healthy.

Humans are part of an energy pathway which can be demonstrated in the following diagram.

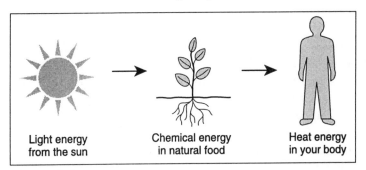

Figure 8.2

No small wonder then that so many cultures have worshipped the sun, as it is truly the giver of life on this planet.

Much of the food we eat, however, is removed from this energy pathway and processed in a factory. Unnatural chemicals are often added, such as flavourings, colourings or preservatives. The food is depleted of its natural energy, it is 'dead' so to speak. It is also toxic for the body due to the presence of these additives and this increases the work of elimination from the body.

The message is simple—the closer your food is to Nature, the higher its energy content and the healthier your body will be.

Water
Water is the body's single most important nutrient. Approximately 60% of the human body consists of water, so we should remember to drink lots of it daily. It is recommended that a 50 kg woman should drink

approximately 1–1½ litres daily. A 70 kg man should consume 1½–2 litres per day.

While these quantities are just guidelines, the most important thing is to listen to your own body. When you are thirsty, drink water—but make sure it's safe water! Filtered or fresh spring water is best, although bottled is better than tap water.

The quality of our water supplies has become a major public health issue. Children seem to know instinctively that tap water is unsuitable for drinking—the odour and taste probably give them instant clues. Many children in modern cities and towns take in the bulk of their fluid requirements from soft drinks rather than water. Soft drinks are composed of carbonated water to which flavourings, colourings and other substances are added. In many cities, tap water is not only foul-tasting and foul-smelling, it also contains chlorine, fluoride, heavy metals and other chemicals which can be potentially harmful to the body. If your pets are not willing to drink it, treat it with suspicion.

Chlorine is used to kill harmful bacteria in the water supply (this is why it's added to swimming pools). But chlorine will also kill some of the 'good' bacteria in the human digestive system. Chlorine has been found to provoke asthmatic attacks and to contribute to arteriosclerosis (hardening of the arteries).

Fluoride is another substance commonly added to the water supply in many countries. While it is intended to prevent tooth decay, fluoride has been shown to damage brain and nerve cells and to cause liver damage. It creates a high incidence of bone fractures as well. Fluoride stimulates bone formation but the bone is often poorly mineralised and therefore more liable to fracture.

When I was a child in Northern Ireland, we lived in the countryside and had a well in our back garden. This was our main source of water for a number of years. Since few chemical insecticides and pesticides were used on the soil in those days, the water was pure and safe to drink. It came straight from Nature. Now, however, reports of the chemical analyses done on the water table in different parts of Europe leave one in no doubt about the damage done to our precious water supplies over the last forty years. As a result, we are forced to consume either filtered water or bottled water.

In the late-1960s, when I was still at school, we went on a school trip to France. I was surprised to see so many French people drinking water from a bottle, as I had never seen bottled water before. Today, bottled water is commonplace the world over. This is a reflection of how *unsafe* our water supplies have become.

In Africa, water is a life-and-death issue. Due to the contamination of the water supply, a significant percentage of children do not make it through their first year of life—many die from gastro-enteritis and other water-borne diseases. A safe water supply is the key to the health of a whole village or community in Africa. Unfortunately, the same is becoming true in Europe. The most basic of all nutrients, water, is now becoming unsafe to drink.

Sugar

The amount of sugar consumed by the average adult and child in the western world is indeed worrying. When shopping in the supermarkets of Europe, it is alarming to see just how many of the foods contain sugar. Most breakfast cereals contain sugar—a bowl of muesli may contain the equivalent of two tablespoons of sugar. Soft drinks also have a high sugar content—Lucozade and Coca Cola contain the equivalent of seven teaspoons of sugar per glass (200 ml)! These examples show how important it is to read the labels on all processed foods. If you wish to know the quantity of any of the constituents of a particular food item, write to the manufacturer.

Refined sugar, like refined flour, is a product of western civilisation. It's an *unnatural* food and so, completely unnecessary in the diet. Worse still, it contributes to ill health. Over 150 years ago, Native American Indians warned of the harmful effects of refined sugar on the body. They observed that the white man ate too many sweet things, which weakened the body. Today, those words are proving to be all too true.

Sugar encourages the growth of a number of bacteria and fungi—it is a wonderful growth medium for these micro-organisms. As a result, a diet rich in sweet things may predispose a person to infections. Sugar consumption is associated with tooth decay, *candidiasis* and mucus production, especially in people predisposed to respiratory problems, such as asthmatics. Many people are now addicted to sugar. As with cigarettes, it can become very difficult to live without it.

In one study by Sanchez et al. (1973), a high intake of sugar was found to have a negative effect on the immune system. These researchers showed that sugar impaired the ability of white blood cells to gobble up and kill bacteria. This research followed the work of an American physician named Dr Sandler, who, while working with victims of the polio epidemic in the late-1940s, became convinced that a high sugar intake made one more susceptible to this disease. The 1973 research supported Dr Sandler's hypothesis, as refined sugar was clearly found to suppress the immune system. Other studies have shown that sugar robs the body of certain nutrients, including zinc (Chapter 9), which is vital for immune function.

The best sugar is always that which is found in Nature, especially in fresh or dried fruits. Raisins, sultanas and dates are excellent sources of sugar and can be used instead of sugar to sweeten breakfast cereal. Many Africans chew on raw cane sugar and do not suffer the health problems that we do in the west. This may be because eating the natural substance supplies the body with minerals such as calcium, whereas eating refined sugar can rob the body of calcium.

Sugar has a detrimental effect on the health of all of us, but most especially on young children who often consume excessive amounts. Many of the children attending my clinic suffer from recurrent infections, asthma and eczema. An alarming number of them are also deficient in various minerals. The first thing I recommend for these children is a reduction in sugar intake. Some are in such a poor state of health that it is necessary to cut out all sugars for a limited period, thereby allowing their young bodies to recover. The benefits of this treatment are almost immediate. There is an increase in both appetite and energy levels. The whole body starts to function better.

Among the adults that I see, there is almost an epidemic of fungal infections, skin rashes and intestinal *candidiasis*. Many of these infections improve when sugar, and foods that contain sugar, are excluded from the diet.

At public talks I am often asked 'Doesn't the body need sugar?' The answer is 'Yes, it does'—but not in the form of unnatural sugars such as glucose, dextrose and sucrose, taken in large quantities on a regular basis. The sugar in fruit and honey—fructose—is natural and much healthier. And remember, starchy foods such as potatoes and rice consist of long chains of glucose molecules. These chains are slowly broken down by the digestive system and glucose is gradually absorbed into the bloodstream.

Look at the two graphs in Figure 8.3. When natural foods containing starch are eaten, the blood sugar level rises gradually (solid line). When this reaches a certain point the pancreas releases insulin and the blood sugar level slowly drops back to normal again. In contrast to this, eating foods

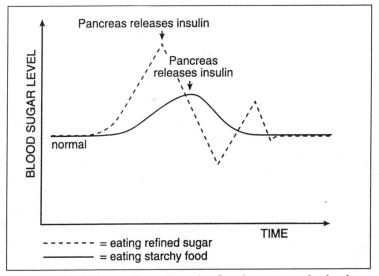

Figure 8.3 Effects of starch and refined sugar on the body

rich in refined sugar (such as sweets) causes high levels of glucose to enter the bloodstream rapidly (dashed line). This puts stress on the pancreas and it is forced to release large quantities of insulin, as too much sugar in the bloodstream can be dangerous (hyperglycaemia).

The ups and downs in the blood sugar level which occur when sugary foods are consumed disturb the body. They put stress on the pancreas and adrenal glands (secrete adrenaline) and can cause the blood sugar level to drop below normal (hypoglycaemia), as shown by the troughs in the graph. Eating sugary foods occasionally does not cause too much difficulty—it is only when the pancreas and adrenal glands are constantly stressed that problems arise. Avoid such difficulties by only eating natural foods and avoiding sugars that have been bleached, chemically refined and rendered harmful to the body.

Processed foods
Nature did not intend us to eat from bottles, tins, jars and packets. The body likes food it can digest and assimilate easily. It likes not only protein, carbohydrate and fat in this form, but also vitamins and minerals. Putting natural foods into a natural system makes sense. Ingesting unnatural chemicals, such as those found in processed foods, does not make sense.

During the 1950s and 1960s, processed foods became part of that dubious package sold to people in the west called 'progress'. The country market was replaced by the supermarket in the belief that bigger was better. Even the supermarkets grew up to become hypermarkets. Remember that the primary aim of the food processing industry is profit, not health! It is encouraging to see that country markets are springing up again and that the availability of organically-grown foods is on the increase. This trend must be encouraged for the sake of ourselves and our children. Put pressure on your local shop/greengrocer to supply organically-grown foods.

The quality of commercially-produced cereals, fruits and

vegetables has declined considerably in the last ten years. A carrot grown in a market garden near a large city is generally of a much poorer quality than a carrot grown in an unspoilt area. Because of economic pressures, chemicals are used in commercial farming and this results in the depletion of the soil itself. A depleted soil produces depleted, poorer-quality vegetables. All the nutrients that a carrot needs must come from the soil. If the goodness of the soil becomes depleted, because too many crops have been grown too quickly, the soil will lack essential minerals and vitamins. When you eat food grown under these circumstances, your body also becomes deprived of certain nutrients, and so the cycle of mineral/vitamin deficiency begins.

The best-quality cereals, fruits and vegetables come from organic farms, that is farms which do not use chemical fertilisers, chemical pesticides or chemical herbicides and which allow time for the soil to replenish itself between crop cycles.

You can now begin to see why it is important to know how and where your fruits and vegetables are grown. If in doubt, grow your own or buy organically-grown produce.

Live yoghurt

If you knew how important it is to consume live yoghurt, you would be eating barrels of it every day! If you want to avoid bowel disease, from constipation through to bowel cancer, eat a carton or two (approximately 100–200 ml) of live yoghurt daily.

WHAT DOES LIVE YOGHURT CONTAIN?

Live yoghurt contains the bacterial cultures *Lactobacillus bulgaricus* and *Streptococcus thermophilus*—these are found in most fermented milk products, including buttermilk. It also contains cultures which are known to be important for bowel function—*Lactobacillus acidophilus* and *Bifidobacterium bifidus* (often shortened to Acidophilus and Bifidus respectively). These two cultures hold the secret to the therapeutic effects of live yoghurt.

Live yoghurt differs from commercial yoghurts in that it is *not* heat-treated after the bacterial cultures are added. Therefore, the live bacterial cultures are able to survive in the intestine and multiply. Most commercial yoghurts are heat-treated, which kills the beneficial live cultures. So, commercial yoghurts do not have the same therapeutic value as yoghurts which have a living culture of Acidophilus and Bifidus.

WHY IS IT BENEFICIAL TO TAKE LIVE YOGHURT?

The skin, the digestive tract (from mouth to anus) and the vagina in females, are colonised by billions of bacteria which are essential for the proper functioning of these organs. In medical terms, these billions of bacteria are referred to as the body's *bacterial flora*. They live both on our skin and inside us. The greatest number of bacteria are found in the digestive tract, where up to 500 different species reside. Collectively, these bacteria are referred to as the *intestinal flora*. The intestinal flora are responsible for numerous important activities, some of which are closely linked to immune function, nutritional status and detoxification of the body.

The quality of our intestinal flora is determined by the balance between the various species of bacteria. Each species keeps the others in check, preventing the overgrowth of any one species. This ecological balance can be disturbed by certain factors such as diet, chronic stress, surgery, major temperature changes and drugs (such as antibiotics). If, for example, the body's bacterial flora are partly destroyed by taking an antibiotic, harmful bacteria can replace the 'good' bacteria which have been destroyed. Certain antibiotics, like amoxycillin, can upset the bacterial flora of the bowel and vagina. In both of these regions, a yeast infection called thrush, which is caused by *Candida albicans*, can develop. A thrush infection is more apparent in the vagina as a visible discharge; it is less apparent in the bowel, as little or no symptoms are present initially.

In a healthy person, 'good' bacteria such as those found in live yoghurt (Acidophilus and Bifidus) produce acids like lactic acid, which keep the environment around them acidic. Harmful bacteria and yeast, such as those responsible for thrush, cannot grow in an acidic environment. They can only grow when the environment becomes less acidic. This can happen when certain drugs are taken (antibiotics and the contraceptive pill in particular). These drugs alter the natural bacterial flora lining the digestive and genital tracts which can result in a chronic infection of these organs with harmful bacteria, yeast or fungi.

'Good' bacteria play a very important role in digestion. For example, the higher the percentage of these 'good' bacteria in the digestive tract, the more peristalsis (natural contractions of the bowel) is stimulated. Peristalsis flushes out waste material in the stool.

The nature of the bacterial population in the intestine has been shown to have a greater effect on bowel habit than the addition of dietary fibre. The medical profession has latched onto bran as the most important dietary factor in the management of many bowel problems. However, while I was still a medical student, the link between cancer of the colon and disturbances in the bacterial population of the bowel had already been clearly established.

A healthy bacterial flora in the intestine has quite a few other beneficial effects. Let's look more closely at some of these.

1. Effects of the intestinal flora on colon cancer

Many studies have shown that the incidence of colon cancer is very low among vegetarians but high among meat eaters. Stool samples from strict vegetarians had a significantly higher population of lactobacilli (*Lactobacillus acidophilus*) —the good guys! Eating meat favoured an increase in putrefactive bacteria such as the bacteriodes (the bad guys) and a decrease in lactobacilli (the good guys). These putrefactive bacteria have the potential to produce chemicals (e.g. toxic amines) which can damage the lining of the colon, ultimately forming a cancerous growth. Since lactobacilli protect against this, it is important to take them on a daily basis as a preventative measure against colon cancer.

It has also been demonstrated that 'good' bacteria are important during the treatment of colon cancer. Neumeister (1969) showed that supplements of the two bacteria found in live yoghurt—*Lactobacillus acidophilus* and *Bifidobacterium bifidus*—taken during irradiation therapy reduced the side-effects of this therapy (e.g. diarrhoea) from 61% to 21%. Other studies have confirmed this, so I recommend the use of a beneficial bacterial culture (such as live yoghurt) during radiotherapy and chemotherapy in the treatment of cancer.

2. The intestinal flora and calcium absorption
The absorption of calcium across the wall of the intestine into the bloodstream is enhanced by a healthy intestinal flora. As explained earlier, 'good' bacteria in the intestine produce acids, such as lactic acid. Calcium absorption is enhanced in an acidic environment. This is particularly important when osteoporosis[6] may be a concern, especially in post-menopausal women who do not exercise much and who have a low calcium content in their diet. Taking live yoghurt daily can help calcium absorption and help to prevent osteoporosis.

3. The intestinal flora and cholesterol
Several studies have shown that the consumption of 'good' bacteria, such as Acidophilus, causes a reduction in serum cholesterol levels (Mann and Spoerry, 1974; Mann, 1977). In addition, feeding a milk formula supplemented with lactobacilli to infants was shown to result in lower levels of blood cholesterol than when milk without lactobacilli was fed to them. Similar observations were reported on piglets that were fed a high cholesterol diet.

These studies verify that taking 'good' bacteria, such as those found in live yoghurt, can reduce the level of blood cholesterol and therefore reduce the risk of heart disease.

4. The intestinal flora and constipation/diarrhoea
Both constipation and diarrhoea can be treated with live

6 Osteoporosis occurs when calcium leaks out of the bones, making them more prone to fracture.

yoghurt. Numerous medical researchers have shown the beneficial effects of lactobacilli on bowel movements, either as live yoghurt or in the form of freeze-dried capsules.

Regular bowel movements are important for everyone, but are even more essential in old age. The consumption of live yoghurt by the elderly population has benefits not only for the bowel but also for the body in general. The calcium in yoghurt is a protection against osteoporosis.

Diarrhoea is a frequent problem for people who are travelling. Travellers often suffer from all kinds of gastro-intestinal problems, particularly infections like gastro-enteritis, which can turn into a long-lasting infection. Taking lactobacilli prior to and during a holiday can protect from diseases caused by intestinal pathogens.

5. The intestinal flora and antibiotic therapy

Therapy with any antibiotic (particularly broad-spectrum antibiotics such as amoxycillin, tetracycline and ampicillin) and the long-term use of antibiotics (as in the treatment of acne) are liable to alter the balance of the intestinal flora. Very strong antibiotics such as clindamycin and lincomycin may cause drastic changes. Taking antibiotics orally often causes gastro-intestinal disturbances, especially in young children. Many complain of vague symptoms such as nausea, dull ache and a sickly feeling all over the abdomen. Others have symptoms such as diarrhoea (probably the most common side-effect of antibiotic therapy), flatulence, bloating and loss of appetite. Long-term problems can range from allergies, recurrent infections and irritable bowel syndrome, to more serious problems such as chronic *candidiasis* (intestinal thrush), diabetes and liver damage.

Because of the increased susceptibility to illness after antibiotic therapy, it is very important to re-establish the normal intestinal flora as soon as possible. In the 1950s, doctors used to advise their patients to use a bacterial culture while taking a course of antibiotics. Today, that practice has stopped even though many more antibiotics are being taken, with stronger ones being used much more commonly.

When on a course of antibiotics, take a supplement of

'good' bacteria, preferably Acidophilus in combination with Bifidus. This will protect you against many gastro-intestinal side-effects.

6. *The intestinal flora produce vitamins essential for well-being*

When a live culture of lactobacilli is present, as in fermented milk products like live yoghurt, there is a huge increase in the levels of folic acid and most B vitamins. This has been demonstrated scientifically. What remains in doubt is how much of these vitamins are actually absorbed across the wall of the intestine and therefore used in the body.

Lactobacilli in the intestine manufacture vitamin K_2. This vitamin is required for the formation of substances necessary for the clotting of blood in the liver. Hence the body is dependent on bacteria in the intestine to manufacture enough vitamin K_2 to ensure normal blood clotting. A vitamin K deficiency can result in nose bleeds, excessive bruising, blood in the urine (haematuria) and excessive menstrual blood loss. Fortunately, some vitamin K is present in green vegetables as vitamin K_1. So, even if the bacterial flora in the bowel are disturbed, you may not develop a vitamin K deficiency if you are eating plenty of green vegetables.

In hospitals, it is common to see a vitamin K deficiency in new-born infants as they have no lactobacilli in the intestine to synthesise this vitamin. Most hospitals give babies 1 mg of vitamin K at birth as a prophylactic measure against the development of spontaneous bleeding—further testimony to the importance of a healthy bacterial population in the digestive tract.

Among the primitive peoples that I have spent time with —the Fulani of West Africa, the Masai of East Africa, the Bushmen of Southern Africa, and the Zulus, Sotho and Xhosa of South Africa—I have been interested to observe that all use curded (fermented) milk. Most groups of people, including the Irish, have used or still use fermented milk as live yoghurt, curded milk, buttermilk and so forth. You are now learning why! The wisdom of these old ways is now being revealed through science.

7. A healthy intestinal flora can prevent bowel infections

There is now conclusive scientific evidence to show that lactobacilli produce substances which inhibit the growth of disease-causing organisms (pathogens). The use of lactobacilli as dietary supplements has been found to alleviate intestinal infections in humans as well as animals (Shahani and Ayebo, 1980). Lactobacilli produce *biocines* which can kill off invading pathogens or inhibit their growth. *Lactobacillus acidophilus* is one species of lactobacilli and it produces several of these substances such as acidophilin, lactocidin and acidolin (Hamdan et al., 1973).

8. The intestinal flora stimulates the immune system

The bacterial population of the intestine is constantly changing—it is a dynamic population, not a static one. The body must react to these changes—the immune system in particular must respond. Hence, changes in the bacterial flora stimulate the immune system and so increase the body's resistance. This strong immune effect of a changing flora is essential if the body is to distinguish between friendly bacteria and harmful ones. This is how the intestinal flora help your immune system.

These are just some of the benefits of taking a bacterial supplement. I recommend taking a daily supplement, especially if you have bowel problems or if you are taking a course of antibiotics.

Other bacterial supplements (apart from live yoghurt)

For the most part, live yoghurt is made from cows' milk, although it can also be made from sheep's or goats' milk. Anyone who does not want to take fermented milk in the form of live yoghurt can take a bacterial supplement in the form of freeze-dried capsules instead. These capsules contain the beneficial bacteria *Lactobacillus acidophilus* either by itself, or in combination with other bacteria such as

Bifidobacterium bifidus. These tablets are sold in most health food shops and pharmacies under the trade names Acidophilus, Biodophilus and Multidophilus. While these tablets are excellent, I always prefer to recommend what Nature provides, which is fermented milk. However, I am aware that some people, particularly children, find it difficult to take live yoghurt, while others are allergic to cows' milk. For them, the freeze-dried capsules are excellent alternatives. If using capsules, keep them in a cool place and remember, once opened, capsules only last for about three weeks so they should be replaced after this time.

There are a few diet-related factors to consider when using a bacterial supplement. Bacteria are sensitive to temperature, so try not to take either very cold or very hot food/drinks along with the supplement. It is also best to combine food correctly when using a supplement—for example, do not combine protein and starchy foods (bread, potatoes, rice, pasta) in the same meal. If foods are combined incorrectly, the food is delayed in the stomach for too long. This increases the exposure of the bacterial supplement to stomach acid which can kill all of the bacteria. The faster the bacterial supplement gets out of the stomach and into the small intestine, the greater the number of bacteria that will survive.

WHEY

> *Little Miss Muffet*
> *Sat on a tuffet,*
> *Eating her curds and whey . . .*

The curds that Little Miss Muffet ate would have contained live bacterial cultures similar to those in live yoghurt. Whey is a by-product in the manufacture of cheese. When the fat and protein are removed from milk to make cheese, what remains is called whey. It contains a high concentration of lactic acid and milk enzymes. Acids, such as lactic acid, maintain a low pH in the bowel and kill off any overgrowth of unhealthy bacteria and fungi; the low pH also stimulates peristalsis, allowing for regular bowel motions.

Being acidic, whey is a natural antiseptic. It is an excellent remedy for sore throats and catarrh of the respiratory tract. Whey cures were famous throughout Europe in the last century and many, including royalty, used to visit the health spas of Switzerland to undergo a 'whey cure'. These were used to treat a whole range of bowel disorders (from constipation to pancreatic problems), hormonal problems, obesity, and circulatory problems such as blocked arteries.

Like live yoghurt, whey should be taken on a regular basis, especially if there are bowel problems such as flatulence, constipation, alteration in the bowel habit, alteration in the bacterial population, diverticulitis, colitis, and chronic bowel infections. Over the last six years, I have treated these intestinal disorders and can support what the Swiss doctors have been saying for many years about the importance of whey and yoghurt.

If taking whey internally, put anything from a teaspoonful to a tablespoonful in a glass of water and take with each meal. This will regulate the secretion of acid from the stomach as well as assisting the colon. Since whey is a by-product of cheese-making, it can be obtained from farms where cheese is manufactured. It can also be obtained commercially in some health food shops. Molkosan is a product produced by Dr Alfred Vogel, the famous Swiss naturopath, and it is an excellent source of whey.

Summary

I knew very little about nutrition on leaving medical school. Most of what I've learned since then has been from courses on natural medicine, mainly in Austria. I once took nutrition to be unimportant and less exciting than pharmacology (the use of drugs). Today, however, I realise that apart from breathing, the most important thing we do every day is eat. What we put into our bodies is of the utmost importance. Nutrition should occupy a prime place in medical education.

Drinking sufficient water every day as well as cutting down on, or cutting out, sugary and processed foods will benefit your health tremendously.

Live yoghurt differs significantly from commercial yoghurt

in that it is not heat-treated after the live bacterial cultures are added to the milk. As a result, the helpful bacteria, especially *L. acidophilus* and *B. bifidus*, survive and can multiply in the bowel.

The benefits of having a high concentration of helpful bacteria in the bowel are numerous. These include: improved digestion; improved immunity; reduced risk of bowel disease, especially cancer; improved absorption of important nutrients, such as calcium; and lower cholesterol levels in the blood.

Again, let me emphasise the importance of taking live yoghurt when taking antibiotics, when undergoing chemotherapy or radiotherapy, or when suffering from constipation, colitis, diverticulitis and intestinal polyps. Bowel function, which is the key to good health, is assisted tremendously by the daily use of live yoghurt and whey. Many of my patients have benefited from this alone, and have not required other medication.

Remember—healthy food and water are the best medicines available!

CASE HISTORY 9

Jane — Intestinal problems

A number of my patients with bowel problems have experienced great relief from using bacterial supplements. Jane is a good example of one of these patients. She came to me complaining of diarrhoea alternating with periods of constipation, bloating, and abdominal cramps, especially after eating. She told me her husband would complain that her tummy was 'rumbling and grumbling' all night long. She herself was very aware of the gurgling noises in her intestine and it was a source of great embarrassment to her.

Jane had been on the contraceptive pill continuously for five years. She had also taken tetracycline and doxycycline during the past year, each for three months, as treatment for acne.

I suspected a disturbance of the intestinal flora for three

reasons: her symptoms; the use of two broad-spectrum antibiotics, both of which are known to cause gross disturbance of the intestinal flora; and her use of the contraceptive pill, which is also known to upset the intestinal flora. Laboratory tests revealed a low percentage of lactobacilli in the stool. Her dietary history also revealed that she had a high intake of processed foods and a very low intake of fresh vegetables and fruit, and that she combined foods incorrectly.

I taught Jane simple food combining, asked her to increase her intake of fresh fruit and vegetables and recommended a bacterial supplement—live yoghurt in this case. She was to take this daily over a three-month period, as well as one tablespoon of whey in a glass of water with each meal. With these simple measures, her bowel habits returned to normal and the bloating and cramps disappeared. In Jane's case, no medicine was necessary, which surprised even me, as I suspected from her initial visit that I would have to use Tetracycline injeel, a homeopathic medicine used to undo the harmful effects of tetracycline in the body. Jane proved the point that simple measures often work best if given time, and that good food is often the best medicine of all.

9 Nutritional Supplements

Nutritional supplements in the form of vitamins and minerals are becoming increasingly important, even if your diet is healthy and well balanced. Since the soil in which our food is grown may be depleted in nutrients, this shortage can be carried all the way through the food chain.

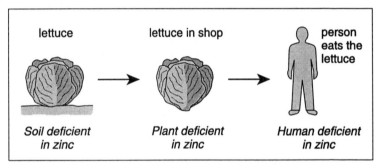

Figure 9.1 Mineral deficiencies in soil can affect your health (e.g. zinc)

This diagram illustrates the point well. It also helps me explain to patients the reason why they are deficient in certain nutrients. For example, a recent analysis carried out on a sample of oranges found that they contained negligible amounts of vitamin C—a rather alarming finding. Organically-grown foods are less likely to have these problems. Firstly, the soil in which they are grown has not been robbed of all its goodness, i.e. it has not been over-exploited. Secondly, only natural fertilisers, such as dung, are used to supplement the soil.

If you need to take a mineral or vitamin supplement, it is

best to use a multi-mineral or multi-vitamin supplement.

Vitamin C
This is the vitamin that first stirred my interest in nutritional medicine. In the early 1970s, I was studying at Trinity College, Dublin. At that time, the Pathology Department was looking at the effect of viral infections on the levels of vitamin C in white blood cells. Students were paid a nominal amount—£1 I think—to give blood samples for analysis if they happened to have a cold. The results of the study confirmed the findings of other researchers, namely that vitamin C is important for the proper functioning of white blood cells.

Dr Linus Pauling, the Nobel Prize laureate, had been preaching the benefits of vitamin C for years—he himself took large doses of it daily. His research, as well as that of others, showed that people taking 200–1000 mg of vitamin C daily had fewer colds than those who were given a placebo (an inactive tablet).

In 1965, the American biochemist Irwin Stone conducted research into the biochemical effects of vitamin C in the body. On the basis of his findings he proposed that the optimum daily intake of vitamin C, for the maintenance of good health, was 1000–5000 mg.

Both Dr Pauling and Dr Stone found it interesting that the American Academy of Sciences recommends a vitamin C intake of 60 mg daily for humans, but 2000 mg per day for laboratory monkeys. In addition, it is known that a gorilla in the wild obtains up to 5000 mg of vitamin C per day in its diet. Clearly we humans need much higher levels of vitamin C than are being recommended at present.

Dr Robert Cathcart, the orthopaedic surgeon renowned for designing the artificial hip, has also turned to nutritional medicine—he prescribes massive doses of vitamin C to patients with infections. The results are quite remarkable. He has shown that it is possible to use only high-dose vitamin C, and nothing else, to treat an infection successfully.[7]

---

7 Other studies have shown that serious illnesses, such as viral meningitis and viral pneumonia, can be treated successfully using high-dose vitamin C alone (Klenner, 1948 and 1951).

There is now a huge body of scientific evidence to show that vitamin C is not only anti-viral and antibacterial, but that it also enhances aspects of a person's immunity, including white cell function, antibody levels and thymus gland function. This evidence clearly indicates that there is a positive role for vitamin C both in treating an infection and in preventing a recurrence. I generally recommend vitamin C doses of 8000–10,000 mg (or higher) in the treatment of an existing infection, and a lower maintenance dose of 2000–4000 mg to prevent recurrence in susceptible patients. Since this vitamin is not stored in the body, there is no concern about overloading the body with too much.

DAILY REQUIREMENTS

Daily requirements for vitamin C vary considerably, not only between individuals, but also within the same individual from day to day. For example, when you are healthy and feeling well, your daily requirement may be as low as 200 mg. But if you become stressed for any reason, it may rise to 1000 mg. In addition, if you are in the early stages of developing an infection, your daily requirement may be even higher, as much as 3000 mg. It has been noted that children who receive a vaccination have much higher vitamin C requirements.

The body's requirements for vitamin C increase in the following situations: pregnancy, stress, surgery, infections, and trauma. On average, however, the daily vitamin C requirement has been estimated biochemically as being between 1000 mg and 5000 mg. The body knows what it needs, so any excess is excreted via the kidneys.

THE EVIDENCE — VITAMIN C WORKS

In the U.S. in 1977, the National Cancer Institute stated publicly that 60% of cancers in women and 40% of cancers in men appear to be related to diet. Yet this same institution spends approximately 1% of its budget on nutritional research. This is clear testimony that nutrition is considered of little importance in the prevention and treatment of cancer, as well as other diseases, within conventional medical circles.

The under-use of vitamin C is one example of the prevailing attitude within the medical profession, that nutrition is not *real* medicine.

Several studies have shown decreased levels of vitamin C in the blood of patients with infections. The levels decreased further as the infection progressed. The more severe the infection, the lower the level of vitamin C. Taking vitamin C in large doses prevents the infection from developing in the first instance, it shortens the duration of the infection and it reduces the severity of the disease. There is considerable scientific evidence now to support these claims (see bibliography). One example I find particularly interesting is discussed in Dr Kalokerinos' book, *Every Second Child*. It emphasises the life-and-death importance of vitamin C.

In the 1960s, while working in rural Australia, Dr Kalokerinos observed that many Aboriginal children and some European children died spontaneously, even though they only had minor symptoms, such as a runny nose and a mild cough. He postulated that these children, who died from what is now called cot death (Sudden Infant Death Syndrome) were suffering from vitamin C deficiency. The basis for this hypothesis was his clinical experience—when these children were dying and not responding to antibiotics or other life-saving drugs, an injection of vitamin C led to a very dramatic and instant recovery. This happened so many times that he soon realised that these children were suffering from scurvy. (The medical profession in Australia treated his work with disbelief. Remember that most doctors are not taught about the clinical use of vitamins and minerals at medical school.)

Dr Kalokerinos also noticed that when normal childhood vaccines (BCG, polio, diphtheria, pertussis and tetanus) were given to Aboriginal children, every second child died. He believed that these children had a low immunity as a result of a poor diet—they lived on processed foods, white sugar, white bread, and ate little or no fresh fruit and vegetables. Dr Kalokerinos then started giving each child vitamin C in a dose of 100 mg per day per month of age—a 3-month-old child received 300 mg daily, a 4-month-old child 400 mg daily, and so on. When they were later immunised, none of these children died. Because this work has been validated by many others, a number of doctors in different parts of the world now use similar doses of vitamin C around the time of vaccination.

As a parent, you can protect your child from the potentially damaging effects of vaccination, particularly the MMR vaccine which is surrounded by a great deal of controversy. Use the above dosage of vitamin C on the day before, the day of, and the day following vaccination. This applies to any vaccine given in the first two years of life. For older children, especially with the MMR vaccine, use higher doses of vitamin C, and for a longer period.

The studies performed over the years by Dr Linus Pauling attest to the benefits of vitamin C in the treatment of viral infections such as the common cold, as well as bacterial infections. In one study, a concentration of 1 mg of vitamin C per decilitre of growth medium prevented the growth of the bacterium that causes tuberculosis. At higher concentrations (greater than 1 mg per decilitre of growth medium), vitamin C has been shown to neutralise the toxins associated with diphtheria, tetanus and staphylococcus.

The effectiveness of vitamin C in cancer treatment was the subject of a conference in 1991, organised by the National Cancer Institute in America. This conference was helpful in informing doctors and patients alike of the benefits of taking vitamin C on a daily basis. It also represented a change of heart within the medical profession—recognition that perhaps nutritional medicine had something important to add, something which doctors could no longer afford to ignore.

How vitamin C works

Vitamin C is essential for the activity of white blood cells. White blood cells are like soldiers in the body—they fight off invading pathogens such as viruses, bacteria or fungi. With high levels of vitamin C, these white blood cells become much more active. Their killing ability becomes more effective.

Various research projects have addressed the role of vitamin C in increasing interferon levels (interferon is an anti-viral substance produced in the body), increasing antibody levels in the bloodstream, and boosting the activity of the thymus gland (a gland which plays a very important part in the immune system). Many doctors and researchers use very high doses of vitamin C in the treatment of AIDS, cancer, and other diseases, where boosting the immune function is of primary importance.

So, vitamin C has a positive effect on different parts of the immune system, making it easier for the body to deal with infection.

THE BEST FORM OF VITAMIN C

If you are taking large amounts of vitamin C it is best to take the acid form, ascorbic acid, as this is more readily absorbed into the bloodstream. However, pure ascorbic acid has quite a low pH and this can cause irritation to the stomach, especially among older people. In such instances, the salt, sodium ascorbate or calcium ascorbate, can be taken instead. Bear in mind that this is less well absorbed by the body and so less is available for the white blood cells to use. A good compromise would be to use a 50:50 mixture of the salt and the acid.

If taking doses greater than 1000 mg per day, it is easier to take vitamin C in powdered form. For smaller doses and children's doses, the commercial tablets available in most chemists/pharmacies are perfectly fine.

At the talks and seminars that I give, I am often asked about the risk of developing kidney stones through taking very high doses of vitamin C. Research in this area (Hoffer, 1985) indicates that there is very little risk of this happening in the majority of people. In fact, it is only those individuals who are prone to the development of kidney stones in the first place, who need to take care. It is recommended that susceptible individuals should use magnesium and pyridoxine to minimise this risk further.

1. It protects against arthritis and other degenerative diseases
Vitamin C is an excellent anti-oxidant so it protects against the onset of chronic degenerative diseases, such as arthritis.

2. It counteracts asthma
There is now mounting evidence to suggest that many asthmatics have reduced levels of vitamin C. One study indicated that a 500 mg dose of vitamin C taken ninety minutes before vigorous exercise lessens bronchial spasms or wheezing in some patients.

Vitamin C also has a role to play in assisting patients with allergies. It prevents the release of histamine (which causes many of the symptoms associated with allergies) by stabilising the membrane of basophils (a type of white blood cell). Since children and adults with asthma are sometimes prone to infections, it makes good sense to recommend vitamin C to these patients, as it will help prevent infections and reduce allergy-type symptoms. Although I do not suffer from any of the above conditions myself, I still take 1000 mg of vitamin C every day.

3. It prevents cancer
The role of vitamin C in cancer prevention is now attracting a lot of attention, particularly with regard to cancers of the stomach and oesophagus. Vitamin C also seems to have a protective effect against cervical dysplasia (precursor to cancer of the cervix). One study has shown that women whose daily intake of vitamin C is less than 90 mg have a 2.5-times greater risk of developing this pre-cancerous change in the cervix, than women whose intake is greater than 90 mg per day. Apparently up to 40% of women in the U.S. have daily vitamin C intakes of less than 70 mg. More recent work has just confirmed this link between low blood levels of vitamin C and pre-cancer and cancer of the cervix. There is also medical evidence to suggest that vitamin C can suppress the growth of human leukaemia cells in culture.

During his lifetime, Linus Pauling examined and documented the beneficial role of vitamin C in the prevention of cancer, as well as the positive effects it has in treating and preventing infections. The medical profession has consistently chosen to ignore his findings and continues to downplay the role of nutrition and nutritional supplements in human health. Hopefully, this is about to change.

SUMMARY
Vitamin C is very important in the treatment of infections, as well as in their prevention. It stimulates the activity of white blood cells and many other parts of the immune system. I recommend a daily dose of 1000–2000 mg in adults, for preventative purposes, and slightly lower doses in children, depending on age and body weight. I also recommend its use in children at the time of vaccination and in patients with degenerative diseases, such as arthritis and cancer. It is especially important for both children and adults with allergic conditions such as asthma.

Zinc — a vital trace element

In addition to protein, fat and carbohydrate, a balanced diet also requires the intake of minerals. The minerals that our bodies need are divided into two groups—those required in amounts greater than 100 mg daily (we call these minerals), and those required in amounts much smaller than 100 mg daily (we call these trace elements). Zinc belongs to the latter group.

In clinical practice, I have found that trace element deficiencies are much more common than vitamin deficiencies (apart from vitamin C, as most of us have some degree of vitamin C deficiency). Of the trace elements, zinc deficiency is one of the most common. It is also the one most studied by medical scientists because of its role in infections and immunity.

Those more prone to mineral and trace element deficiencies include the elderly, pregnant women, vegetarians, patients on certain drugs (e.g. diuretics), patients with bowel problems (especially where absorption is impaired as in coeliac disease, or where there are intestinal parasites), and patients on intravenous feeding.

In my own practice, a number of children are showing up as marginally zinc deficient, especially those with recurrent infections. A few are actually moderately zinc deficient, even though they are on a supposedly healthy diet. Even mild zinc deficiency can have enormous repercussions on a person's health. This is because more than two hundred enzymes require this trace element for their activity, i.e. many chemical reactions in the body need zinc. So a zinc deficiency can affect a wide number of important reactions in the body. Signs of zinc deficiency include growth retardation, poor appetite, mental lethargy and under-functioning of the sex glands, as well as increased susceptibility to infections. If your child has a poor appetite, always suspect a zinc deficiency.

ZINC AND THE IMMUNE SYSTEM

Zinc is now firmly established as a major protector of the immune system and an important disease fighter. It has been clearly established that zinc is essential for cell-mediated immunity. Take the case of the Dutch Freisian cattle (the A46 mutant strain) with a defect in their absorption of zinc—these cattle have an increased susceptibility to infection and die early. They have been shown to have impaired cellular immunity, which is treated by using a zinc supplement.

There is a rare but similar disorder which affects humans called *Acrodermatitis enteropathica*. People with this disorder are also more susceptible to infections and die young. Again the condition is treatable with zinc. These patients have defects in the immune activity of their white blood cells, as well as in other parts of their immune system.

Research has shown a definite decrease in the number of circulating T-lymphocytes, which fight infection, in patients who are over the age of seventy, one of the groups at risk of recurrent infections. It is now being suggested that one of the reasons why the immune system becomes weaker with age may be because zinc levels are lower. Other studies have shown that patients with AIDS have significantly lower blood levels of zinc when compared to a control group. This suggests a role for zinc supplementation in these patients.

The recommended intake of zinc is 15 mg daily for adults and 10 mg for children. The best dietary sources are whole grain cereals, legumes and meats. Oysters also have very high levels of zinc.

Our ability to absorb zinc decreases with age. Fibre, iron and calcium also diminish the amount of zinc that we are able to absorb. Too much fibre in the diet can reduce the absorption of zinc across the bowel wall into the bloodstream. Too much iron and calcium in the diet can compete with zinc for absorption and reduce its uptake into the body.

I recommend a minimum daily intake of 10–15 mg in children and double this dosage for adults, especially where there is a history of recurrent infections. This is more than the RDA[8], but it is necessary if one is to correct the deficiency quickly and reduce the incidence of infection. I normally recommend zinc supplementation for a three-month period and then reassess the situation.

IS ZINC SUPPLEMENTATION SAFE?

There are no adverse effects associated with low-dose zinc supplementation. Megadoses of zinc, however, in the order of 300 mg daily, may have a negative effect on the immune system, so correct dosage is important. In one particular study, where eleven men took 150 mg of zinc twice a day for six weeks, there was a significant reduction in their immune function (Chandra, 1984). Since zinc competes with copper for absorption across the bowel wall, high doses of zinc could create a deficiency of copper. So, if you are taking a high-dose zinc supplement (i.e. more than the doses I've suggested above) it would be wise to include some copper in the supplementation schedule. A copper dosage which is one-tenth of the zinc dosage should be sufficient. In other words, if taking 50 mg of zinc daily, then take 5 mg of copper with it.

---

[8] RDA: Recommended Daily Allowance as defined by medical scientists.

SUMMARY
Zinc is important in many chemical reactions within the body. Even a mild deficiency can have a significant effect, especially on the immune system. Research has shown a positive role for zinc in protecting the immune system and in fighting disease, especially viral infections where little can be done using conventional medicine.

Foods rich in zinc include oysters, whole grain cereals and legumes. Supplementation is recommended for people who are susceptible to infections, but do not take very high doses of zinc, i.e. over 50 mg daily.

Personal note

During my years in Africa, I noticed that many of the children I examined, with both minor and serious infections, had liver tenderness. I assumed this was due to a viral infection as there are a number of viruses which can affect the lymph glands, liver and spleen. (A good example of this is the Epstein–Barr virus which is associated with glandular fever.) Even after recovery, some of these children still experienced liver tenderness.

While practising in Ireland during the last five years, I have treated numerous children with allergies, diabetes, recurrent infections and asthma. Liver tenderness was an occasional finding in some of these children, but certainly less common than in African children. However, the children in Ireland exhibited the same persistence of liver tenderness even after recovery. Assuming that this may have been viral, I used anti-viral medicines. I had learned a few tricks by then about how to treat viral infections, how to boost the immune system and how to assist the liver in repairing itself. To my surprise, my treatment did not work.

I then decided to try the wonderful herb, Milk Thistle (*Silybum marianum*) to help liver function. In many cases, this did not work either, although it did in a few. I could not explain this, so did not persist in using Milk Thistle either.

Then I read Dr Kalokerinos' book, *Every Second Child*, which describes his investigation into vitamin C deficiencies in Aboriginal children. Dr Kalokerinos' work made me wonder whether the problem which I could not solve might be due to zinc deficiency. Here is what led me to this conclusion.

Dr Kalokerinos had discovered liver tenderness in numerous sick children brought to his hospital, many of whom were dying from apparently minor infections. Post-mortems revealed that all organs were normal, except the liver, which showed yellow patches of fat on the surface. Moreover, in most cases of cot death (sudden infant death syndrome), the state pathologist could find nothing wrong either. Dr Kalokerinos had to wait many years for an explanation. It came from a most unlikely source, an inorganic chemistry professor at the University of Sydney.

Professor Freeman was interested in the role of zinc in the body's chemistry. He postulated that because many liver enzymes need zinc to function properly, a zinc deficiency could cause liver disturbances, predisposing it to fatty degeneration—the yellow deposits of fat found during post-mortems!

I was very excited when I read this as it was the first time I encountered a possible explanation for my observations. I cannot prove it, but zinc supplementation is now on my treatment plan for these children. I hope there will be positive results to report in years to come. Thank you, Dr Kalokerinos!

Clearly there is much work to be done in the area of vitamin C and zinc deficiencies. This kind of research needs much more public support and people need to be made more aware of the prevalence of these deficiencies.

I hope this chapter has made you more aware of the importance of vitamin and mineral supplements, especially if you are prone to infections. Remember that for many people around the world, it can be a life-and-death issue, as Dr Kalokerinos' work highlighted. Never underestimate the importance of nutrition and nutritional supplements in the maintenance of good health.

10   The Role of Stress

'The physical is merely an expression of the spiritual'

Stress and infections

Stress-related illness has reached epidemic proportions in the western world. In Africa, especially in rural areas, it is virtually non-existent. High blood pressure and heart disease (angina and heart attack) are common in the west, but are very rare among the rural black population of southern Africa. As soon as these people move into towns and cities, however, they begin to show signs of hypertension and heart disease. This seems to indicate that the stresses of modern life can have damaging effects on the body.

During the 1920s, Professor Hans Selye of the University of Prague carried out research into the negative effects of stress on the body. His years of research led him to propose the following model, which explains how chronic stress can affect us.

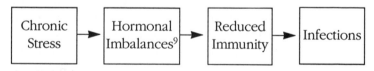

| Chronic Stress | → | Hormonal Imbalances[9] | → | Reduced Immunity | → | Infections |

Figure 10.1

9 When I speak of hormonal imbalances, I am referring to the whole endocrine system, including the hypothalamus, pituitary, thyroid, thymus and adrenal glands, as well as the pancreas, ovaries and testes.

Professor Selye proposed that stress can cause imbalances within the endocrine or hormonal system of the body, which in turn can suppress the immune system. This theory has been supported more recently by other medical researchers. Dr Carl Simonton, for example, who is famous for his pioneering work with cancer patients, proposed that a high percentage of these patients had experienced a period of chronic stress preceding the onset of cancer. Simonton suggested that stress was causing a suppression of the immune system, thereby allowing cancer to develop.

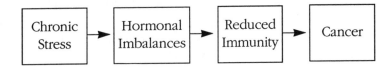

Figure 10.2

From a medical point of view, stress increases output from the adrenal glands, thereby causing a rise in the levels of adrenaline and cortisone in the body. These hormones can suppress white blood cells and cause the thymus gland (part of the immune system) to shrink. This appears to be the mechanism by which stress affects immunity. The level of immune suppression is proportional to both the duration of stress and the level of stress. In contrast, deep relaxation has a positive effect on immune function. One particular scientific reference has shown that powerful immune-enhancing chemicals are released in the body during periods of deep sleep (Moldofsky et al., 1986). This supports what our common sense tells us—that deep relaxation and good-quality sleep can boost immunity and so counteract the effects of stress.

From this evidence, it is reasonable to suggest that chronic stress, through its negative effect on the immune system, can result in an increased susceptibility to infections and to the development of cancer. Hence, it is important to consider the possibility of stress in anyone who presents with recurrent infections, even children. The next case history exemplifies the strong link between emotional stress and recurrent asthmatic attacks.

André — Severe asthma

André was a young man, twenty-two years of age, when I first met him in South Africa. He had been admitted to hospital ten times in the course of six months with severe asthma. Twice he 'died' in casualty and had to be resuscitated.

When André came to see me, I was alarmed by two things. Firstly, there was the high dosage and the amount of medication which he was taking to control the asthmatic attacks. Secondly, there was the number of hospital admissions. This young man was in difficulty but not just at a physical level. André was not consciously aware of any major emotional stresses in his life when I questioned him. The real story came from his mother at a later date. Prior to being adopted, André had suffered great physical abuse from his biological parents. As a young child, he and his brothers and sisters were locked in cupboards for days at a time. They were starved, beaten and burned with cigarette butts. The children were eventually rescued by social workers and placed in care.

Since André was very young at the time, he was unaware of much of this at a conscious level; the information was locked away in his subconscious. It did, however, trigger a pattern of behaviour when he got into difficulty in a relationship, for example, fighting with his girlfriend. This problem may have triggered memories, deep in his subconscious, about his childhood experiences and his relationship with his biological parents. The turmoil was probably too painful to deal with and triggered a cry for help in the form of an asthmatic attack. The words his adoptive mother used to describe the asthmatic attacks conjured up the image of a 'death wish', like someone who found the emotional pain so difficult to deal with, that they wanted to die.

On further questioning, it transpired that all of André's severe asthmatic attacks were preceded by an argument or disagreement with a loved one—girlfriend, adoptive mother or father. Any threat to these relationships was a threat to his survival.

Using physical medicines may have been helpful to André, but it was apparent that his real need was for help at an emotional level. I am pleased to say that he is now undergoing treatment with a clinical psychologist. He has not seen the inside of a hospital for the last eighteen months and we have been able to reduce most of his conventional medicine. No amount of dietary advice, homeopathy, herbal medicines, vitamins or conventional drugs would have solved André's problems.

This case shows that the interaction between the emotional and physical within all of us must never be underestimated. It also demonstrates the inherent danger of viewing someone as purely a physical body, with physical symptoms, which is exactly what was happening each time André was admitted to hospital.

Everyone with asthma receives the same treatment in hospital, despite the fact that no two people are the same. Each one of us is unique. It is essential that treatment is tailored to the individual, not to a standard protocol learned at medical school. Even though two people may have the same diagnosis, they may need very different treatments to get better. Listening and observing are the best diagnostic tools a doctor can have. These are the keys not only to diagnosis, but also to working out a treatment plan for the individual patient.

This case history suggests a link between one's emotional state and one's physical health. But is it really possible that emotional or mental stress can predispose one to an infection?

STRESS AND THE COMMON COLD

Experiments done at Oxford University in the 1970s showed clearly that people under stress, such as business managers constantly facing deadlines, were much more susceptible to the common cold.

Other research done at Carnegie Mellon University in the U.S. showed that among individuals exposed to one of five common cold viruses, 47% of those under high levels of stress became ill, while only 27% of those experiencing low stress levels became sick. The doctors conducting this study suggested that '... stress is associated with the suppression of a general resistance process ... leaving persons susceptible to infectious agents' (Cohen et al., 1991).

Many other studies confirm the idea that stress is associated with the suppression of different immune processes. How does this happen? It appears that when stress is prolonged, the adrenal glands continue to release adrenaline and cortisone. Prolonged elevation of cortisone can cause destruction of the T-lymphocytes in the thymus gland (the master gland of the immune system). It is believed that this suppression of the thymus can predispose a person to infection.

STRESS AND THE MENTAL STATE

Why do some people who are subjected to high levels of stress get sick while others do not? In Dr Cohen's study, quoted above, 47% of those subject to high stress became ill —but what about the remaining 53% who remained well? Both psychologists and medical scientists have been looking for reasons why people do *not* get infections, even though they are exposed to a virus or bacteria. This work makes very interesting reading and basically supports the idea that the physical state is often a mere reflection of the inner state.

The link between mental state and one's immunity has been the subject of much interest. In 1989, Dr D. Sobel and Dr R. Ornstein wrote a book entitled *Healthy Pleasures* in which they quote details of their research into two groups of people, pessimists and optimists. They showed scientifically that optimists enjoy better immune function than pessimists. Optimists were shown to have higher numbers of one type of T-lymphocyte cell, which stimulate immune function, than of a second type, which suppress immune function. The cells that stimulate immune function are called *helper cells*, while those that suppress immune function are called *suppresser cells*. The higher the number of helper cells, the better one's resistance to infection will be. It's interesting to see that someone's mental state can influence their physical response to infection.

STRESS AND THE EMOTIONAL STATE

Research into the ways in which the emotional state affects one's response to stress ranks *anger* as the single most powerful suppresser of immune function, predisposing a person not only to infection but also to a whole host of other illnesses (Angier, 1990).

Dr Mara Julius of the University of Michigan looked at the effects of deep-seated anger on the health of women over an eighteen-year period. Each woman was asked to complete a questionnaire specifically designed to detect suppressed anger. The most startling aspect of this study was the fact that women with a high score on the questionnaire, i.e. those with high levels of anger, were three times more likely to have died during the study period (eighteen years) than those who had little or no suppressed anger. Many studies now show that anger can contribute to early death, heart disease and a range of other problems.

In the book *Beyond Antibiotics*, Dr Michael Schmidt and co-workers state that 'anger and hostility eat away at the substance of the human psyche. These emotions foster an atmosphere of negativity that clouds every human endeavour. Researchers are increasingly showing a link between anger, hostility and cynicism, and the development of disease and premature death.'

Anyone who has participated in my workshops on stress will already know my opinions on the roles played by anger and fear in human disease. In my practice, I've seen a very close link between ill health and one's emotional state. In my opinion, the main obstacle to good health is suppressed anger. I meet this obstacle on a daily basis. In both Ireland and South Africa, the two countries in which I have spent most of my life, I see suppressed anger as the main obstacle not only to one's physical health but also to one's growth and development as a human being.

In Ireland, physical and sexual abuse are alarmingly common—I myself experienced the intense anger embodied within 'holy' men such as priests and Christian Brothers. I lived in dread of going to school every day of my life. But this is nothing compared to some of the stories my patients have recounted in the last few years. I remember one patient who could remember nothing of her childhood from the age of sixteen back to early childhood—yes, nothing! She could not remember a happy memory, a sad one—nothing! Through therapy, it became apparent that the abuse she had suffered had been so great for so long, that her sole means of coping was to pretend it wasn't happening. The courage this woman has shown in facing this pain, and dealing with it, leaves me in awe.

In South Africa, I observed a much higher level of suppressed anger in the white population than in the black population, despite the fact that the black population has suffered so much more in recent times. I think this probably has a great deal to do with the different social support structures found within these two population groups. In black society, problems are shared within the 'extended family structure'. In contrast to this, problems are seldom discussed in the 'single parent family structure' which exists in white society (South Africa has the highest divorce rate in the world).

I believe that the single biggest advancement that can be made, not just for improving one's immune system but for one's total health and the good of humanity, is the release of anger. In Case History 10, quoted earlier in this chapter, André had a high level of anger which was directed against his biological parents. It was only by releasing this anger that he was able to break the cycle of hospital admissions which had brought him to me in the first place. I could quote many other similar cases but it suffices to say that you should *never underestimate the role of your emotions in determining the state of your physical health.*

Negative emotions have powerful effects on the physical

body, primarily through the immune system. Impaired immune function can result in serious infections, auto-immune diseases, cancer and premature death.

SUMMARY
Stress can act via the immune system, allowing recurrent infections to develop. Some of the most effective ways of counteracting stress are deep relaxation, meditation and good-quality sleep, not forgetting a good diet and adequate supplementation where necessary.

Protecting against stress

In modern society, many people suffer from various forms of chronic stress—job pressure, marital disharmony, financial pressure, time spent in traffic, etc. It is important to become aware of the various stresses in your life and their effects on you. The Holmes and Rahe rating scale is a popular method of measuring stress. Although it is not comprehensive, it is useful to relate this scale to your own life as it will roughly assess the degree of stress you might be experiencing. (It refers only to *social* aspects of your life.)

The Holmes and Rahe Rating Scale — Top twenty events

Rank	Life event	Mean value
1	Death of spouse/partner	100
2	Divorce	73
3	Separation	65
4	Time spent in jail	63
5	Death of a close family member	63
6	Personal illness or injury	53
7	Marriage	50
8	Fired from job	47
9	Reconciliation with partner/spouse	45
10	Retirement	45
11	Change in family member's health	44
12	Pregnancy	40
13	Sexual problems	39

Rank	Life event	Mean value
14	New member in family	39
15	Adjustments at work	39
16	Change in financial status	38
17	Death of a close friend	37
18	Changing jobs	36
19	More arguments with spouse/partner	35
20	Large mortgage	31

Various events are rated numerically, according to their potential for causing disease. A score of 200 or more is considered to be predictive of getting a serious illness.

In addition to learning coping skills, with the help of a professional therapist if necessary, there are other important things you can do to help your physical body cope with stress. These can be discussed under four headings—exercise, relaxation, adrenal gland support and ginseng.

THE ROLE OF EXERCISE
Regular exercise leads to an increased ability to cope with stress by:
- improving heart function—exercise reduces heart rate, improves heart muscle tone and reduces blood pressure;
- reducing the output of adrenaline and cortisone from the adrenal glands in response to stress;
- improving the oxygen uptake of all cells in the body;
- improving self-esteem and feeling of well-being;
- increasing energy.

THE ROLE OF RELAXATION
Deep relaxation is one of the most effective anti-stress measures there is. Only you know which relaxation technique is the most effective for you. It can vary from meditation, progressive relaxation, self-hypnosis, visualisation or yoga, through to fishing, reading and dancing. Do what feels right for you.

When deeply relaxed, certain physiological changes occur in the body. These include:
- a reduced heart rate and lower blood pressure;

- better movement of blood from the peripheries towards the internal organs;
- reduced sweat production;
- better digestion, due to increased secretion of digestive juices;
- shallow, calmer breathing rate.

ADRENAL GLAND SUPPORT

Because chronic stress causes a continual increase in adrenaline and cortisone secretion from the adrenal glands, these glands can become exhausted and can shrink or atrophy. Certain nutritional supplements can help prevent adrenal gland damage—particularly potassium, vitamin C, vitamin B_6, pantothenic acid, zinc and magnesium. Hence, a good vitamin and mineral supplement is important. But check that the supplement contains the above ingredients. Potassium and pantothenic acid are particularly important for adrenal gland support. The following chart lists some foods rich in these two substances.

Potassium	Pantothenic acid
avocado	whole grains
potato	legumes
tomato (raw)	cauliflower
banana	broccoli
melon	tomato (raw)
fish	liver

GINSENG

Ginseng protects the body against the harmful effects of stress and protects against physical and mental fatigue. It is the best herb to take to support adrenal function. There are many studies which testify to ginseng's anti-stress activity. They show how ginseng can assist with extremely stressful conditions, improving mental alertness and athletic performance. It can be taken as a herbal tincture (a liquid extract), in dry form or in homeopathic form. I prefer the dried root which I use as a powder, combining it with liquorice to assist absorption into the bloodstream. Put ¼ teaspoon of powdered ginseng root with an equal amount of liquorice in a cup of water. Bring to the boil and simmer for ten minutes. Drink this two or three times a day.

SUMMARY
To protect your body against the adverse effects of stress take regular exercise, allow for periods of relaxation and use natural substances to support the adrenal glands. These should include a good mineral and vitamin supplement, as well as the herb ginseng.

CASE HISTORY 11

John — Pain in the anal sphincter

John worked abroad in the stock exchange and was back home in Ireland for a short visit. He came to see me complaining of tightness and pain in the anal sphincter which made it difficult to have a bowel motion. This problem was getting progressively worse and he was very worried about it. John had noticed that the condition disappeared when he was on holiday. More recently, he had noticed that he got short bouts of palpitations, lasting only a minute or two, intermittently during the day. He described his job as very stressful, as he was doing several things at any one time. He also had to travel a considerable distance to and from his workplace and was essentially away from home for more than thirteen hours each day.

I explained to him that the muscle lining the bowel wall and the anal sphincter were under the control of the autonomic (or involuntary) part of the nervous system. I can simplify this by calling it the adrenalin/nor-adrenalin system, as adrenalin speeds you up (increases heart rate and blood pressure and decreases peristalsis in the bowel), while nor-adrenalin does the opposite by relaxing you (decreases heart rate and blood pressure and increases bowel activity). In other words, the bowel will function best when you are relaxed. You can't force your bowel to work—it works best without your conscious control.

I treated John by giving him relaxation exercises to do every day. I prescribed ginseng and vitamin B complex as anti-stress medicines and asked him to take up yoga or meditation. He improved a lot physically but more importantly he became aware of what his stressful lifestyle was doing to him and is now seeking a new job. He also became aware of other aspects of his lifestyle, in particular his eating habits and the importance of having sufficient energy to enjoy time with his family.

A wonderful change took place inside this man. Stress can be positive—it can lead you to make meaningful changes in your life.

Treating stress

The treatment of chronic stress, now often called 'stress management', deserves a whole book in itself since it involves deeper issues within ourselves. Very often the changes that are occurring in our lives—a change of job, a new relationship, a new home—are interpreted as negative and undesirable. But are they? Change is necessary if we are to grow as human beings. Unfortunately, this growth usually only occurs through pain and suffering. These changes 'appear' to be external. Most, however, are generated by the need to change internally; when the external circumstances alter (the break-up of a relationship, separation from loved ones, failure of a business venture, loss of a job), this allows a space to be created in our lives for internal changes to happen. These changes, even though they may be painful as one goes through them, are always for the better. This may be difficult to accept when in the midst of a painful experience. Years later, however, we may be able to see the truth in this.

CASE HISTORY 12

Angela — Breast cancer

Three years ago a woman diagnosed as having breast cancer, with secondaries in the liver and bone, came to see me. On her third visit to my surgery, she said that she was glad she

131

had developed cancer! I had never heard a cancer patient say this kind of thing before, so I asked her what she meant.

She replied, 'Cancer has helped me to see the beauty all around me. I have always loved flowers but I was always too busy to spend time in my garden. I always walked through the front garden on my way to and from work, but I never found time to simply enjoy it. Because I know that I may die at any time, I now walk into the garden, touch the daffodils, smell them, talk to them—I've become aware of their beauty. Slowly, I've become aware of the beauty in trees and animals. I've become aware of the beauty inside people and wish that they could see it themselves. I've also become aware of the beauty within myself.'

This was a remarkable statement from a woman who had a death sentence hanging over her. Although she had initially interpreted the diagnosis of breast cancer as frightening and negative, she had slowly become more aware. She had developed a deep spiritual awareness of the beauty and creation within all of us. Cancer had helped her to see this. Her level of awareness had developed to the point where she was no longer afraid of death.

Stressful events can have a positive aspect but in order to see this we must focus our thoughts and energy on it. Stress, adversity and change are great motivators. They teach us a great deal about ourselves. As a teacher once said to me, 'The only thing you are guaranteed in life is change, and death is merely a form of change.'

André, the young man with severe asthma in Case History 10, underwent a great personal transformation as a result of his condition. A physical, external illness—asthma—precipitated a whole series of internal changes which were painful and difficult. Today, he has a much greater understanding of himself—and others.

Stress precipitates a need to seek help—from a doctor, a psychologist, a counsellor, even a friend. This sets off a sequence of events which usually result in an inner growth, often in the form of a greater awareness about ourselves and everything going on around us.

At the stress management courses I run, in conjunction with other therapists, we aim to develop a much higher level of awareness in the participants. We try to help people to become more aware, through the experience of novel forms of meditation (Tibetan and Indian), through music and dance, through self-hypnosis and visualisation. We usually run these courses over weekends. This helps people to stop temporarily and remove themselves from their daily routines. We encourage them to focus on the positive side of even the most tragic events in life, and to identify and release the greatest obstacles to human happiness, anger and fear. So much human pain and sickness have their origins in one or both of these feelings. Having the courage to face them and deal with them allows enormous personal growth to take place, to the point where the internal beauty becomes more apparent. We then begin to accept ourselves and to become much more comfortable and at ease.

Stress management addresses the deeper issues and helps us to see the positive side of ourselves. This can only be taught in an experiential way, through doing exercises which enhance awareness. Listening to others speak about their experiences is of little value, since we must experience things for ourselves.

On our weekend courses, we usually begin the day at 7.00 a.m. with a powerful dynamic meditation—this is physically tough, but allows for a deep meditative experience. This lasts for about one hour and is followed by a silent 30-minute walk in the countryside. A light breakfast of water, fruit and herbal tea follows. Throughout the day, we try to create a balance between physical activity, creative activity, periods of silence, relaxation (including swimming and saunas) and other optional activities. After a few days of this, changes begin to occur but these may only become apparent a few days, or even weeks, later.

I believe that this is the only way to approach stress management—through a set of exercises I have developed, through unconditional support and acceptance of the participants, and through creating a safe environment in which everyone can express what they feel deep inside. Only in this way can meaningful changes take place within each of us.

Someone once asked me to state, in one sentence, how to overcome the stresses of modern life. My answer was, 'Be yourself and stop trying to fit someone else's picture of you.' When you are being yourself completely, life works for you and rewards you in ways beyond belief. The purpose of these weekend workshops is to give you the space to be yourself.

Conclusion

The purpose of this book is to show that there are valid and effective ways to treat infections without using antibiotics. Antibiotics have only been produced commercially in the last fifty years—infections were treated in other ways prior to that.

Some of the methods that I use in my practice, with great success, have been mentioned in this book. Hopefully, they will gain more popularity in years to come. The main difficulty I've encountered is the general lack of availability of these preparations in pharmacies and health food shops. In Germany and France, it is very easy to gain access to 'alternative' medicines (homeopathic, herbal, nutritional supplements and mixtures of these) through most pharmacies. Unfortunately, this is not the case in Ireland and the U.K. It is only with your support that this situation will change—ask your local pharmacy to stock some of these medicines.

If you wish to stop using antibiotics and to start using the alternatives that I have suggested, here is some practical advice:

Treating an acute infection
1. Use oral high-dose vitamin C.
For adults, take 10,000 mg daily for two days, then 5000 mg daily for two days, then 2000–3000 mg as a daily maintenance dose for one week.

For children under twelve years, the dosage will vary with age.

Vitamin C in this dosage may be sufficient to control the infection. In some individuals, and where the infection is more serious, even higher doses may be necessary. In a few cases it may be necessary to use vitamin C intravenously. Some doctors in the U.S. have shown that serious infections, such as meningitis and pneumonia, can be treated in this way.

2. Take Echinacea.
Take Echinacea as a herbal extract in liquid form (tincture) at a dose of 2–4 ml, three times daily for seven to ten days.
or
Take Echinacea in homeopathic form, i.e. as a complex remedy. Take 20 drops initially and then 10 drops frequently (up to six times daily) for two days. Then take 10 drops, three times daily, for up to one week after overcoming the infection.

For more serious infections, it is wiser to take Echinacea compositum in ampoule form, either orally or by intra-muscular injection. This medicine can be used twice daily until the symptoms of the infection abate, and then once daily for up to ten days.

If the infection is viral, for example a cold or 'flu, the anti-viral substance Engystol can be taken at the same time in ampoule form along with Echinacea compositum.

3. Drink lots of fluids, rest and be careful about your diet.

These three simple measures can be used by anyone to quickly overcome an infection. However, if you find that the infection is not being controlled by these measures, consult a homeopathic doctor.

Using an antibiotic

If you prefer to use an antibiotic from the outset, or when the previous measures have failed, I suggest you do the following:

1. Make sure the antibiotic is justified.
Have your doctor take a swab or a sputum, a urine or stool sample for laboratory analysis to prove that the infection is bacterial. Antibiotics are only justified when the infection is due to bacteria, not viruses!

2. Take live yoghurt or a bacterial supplement with the antibiotic.
Older doctors used to recommend this when antibiotics first became available in the 1940s and 1950s. The beneficial bacteria in live yoghurt and bacterial supplements will protect against some of the side-effects of antibiotics.

3. Take vitamin C along with the antibiotic.
Some studies have shown that taking vitamin C with an antibiotic results in higher blood levels of the antibiotic, thus making it more effective. Vitamin C will also assist your immunity and help your body to fight the infection.

4. Take Echinacea.
Since some antibiotics can suppress different parts of the immune system, it is wise to take Echinacea as it is renowned for its ability to boost immunity.

Use Echinacea, either in herbal form or as a homeopathic preparation, in the dosage outlined previously. Echinacea in herbal form, when combined with an antibiotic, has been shown to shorten the duration of an infection significantly. Experiments on this have been done in Germany where Echinacea has been recommended as a very useful adjunct to antibiotic therapy.

By taking a bacterial supplement, vitamin C and Echinacea along with an antibiotic, you not only shorten the duration of the infection, you also protect your body against some of the side-effects of antibiotic usage. But remember—only use an antibiotic when it is clearly justified for the treatment of a bacterial infection.

I believe in the old ways of doing things, ways which are simple and natural, ways which are accessible to everyone. Today, medicines are becoming more and more expensive and this makes it difficult for the disadvantaged to gain access to them. Even many natural methods of healing have now become commercially-oriented. Wisdom and a respect for Nature do not sit comfortably beside profit-driven commercial enterprises. Yet the wisdom handed down from generation to generation is vital for our survival. This wisdom, as well as a deep respect for Nature, are evident among the African tribes with whom I have lived. It is also apparent among Native American Indians.

It is encouraging to see an increasing interest in these people and their ways—especially from white westerners, the very people who almost destroyed them! I am pleased to observe and be part of this change, and to see the emergence of a more holistic view, not just of medicine, but of the world as a whole.

It is only by experiencing the negative that we come to value the positive. It is only through pain and suffering that meaningful changes can take place. The changes we are all experiencing are stressful but they are also beautiful. When our children are parents themselves they will benefit from this change, making their world less threatening and stressful.

I hope you have gained something from reading this book and that it has not been too technical. Please write and let me know what your opinions are. Your comments will help me with future editions. I wish you and your loved ones well. May you live happy, healthy lives.

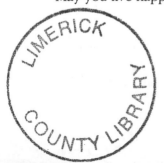

Bibliography

Chapter 1 The History of Antibiotics, pp. 1–11

Chain, E., Florey, H. W., Gardner, A. D. et al., 'Penicillin as a Chemotherapeutic Agent', *The Lancet* Vol. 1, 226–8 (1940).

Cowen, D. L. and Segelman, A. B., *Antibiotics in Historical Perspective*, New Jersey: Merck Sharpe & Dohme 1981.

Fleming, A. (ed.), *Penicillin: Its Practical Application*, London: Butterworth 1946.

Levy, S. B., *The Antibiotic Paradox*, New York: Plenum Press 1992.

McFarlane, G., *Alexander Fleming: The Man and the Myth*, London: Chatto & Windus 1984.

Chapter 2 Bacterial Resistance to Antibiotics, pp. 12–28

Barnes, P. F. and Barrows, S. A., 'Tuberculosis in the 1990s', *Annals of Internal Medicine* Vol. 119(5), 400–410 (1993).

Bloom, B. R. and Murray, C. J., 'Tuberculosis: Commentary on a re-emergent killer', *Science* Vol. 257, 1055–64 (1992).

Chandler, D. and Dugdale, A. E., 'What do patients know about antibiotics?', *British Medical Journal* Vol. 8, 422 (1976).

Holmberg, S. O., Osterholm, M. T., Senger, K. A. and Cohen, M. L., 'Drug resistant *Salmonella* from animals fed anti-microbials', *New England Journal of Medicine* Vol. 10, 311 (1984).

Kitamoto, O. et al., 'On the drug resistance of *Shigella* strains isolated in 1955', *Journal of the Japanese Association for Infectious Diseases* Vol. 30, 403–5 (1956).

Kunin, C. M., 'Resistance to anti-microbial drugs—a worldwide calamity', *Annals of Internal Medicine* Vol. 118(7), 557–61 (1993).

Leclercq, R., Derlott, E., Duval, J. and Courvalin, P., 'Plasmid-mediated resistance to vancomycin and teicoplanin in *Enterococcus faecium*', *New England Journal of Medicine* Vol. 319(3), 157–61 (1988).

Levy, S. B., 'Antibiotic availability and use: consequences to man and his environment', *Journal of Clinical Epidemiology* Vol. 44 Suppl. 2, 835–75 (1991).

Levy, S. B., 'Confronting multi-drug resistance: a role for each of us', *Journal of the American Medical Association* Vol. 269(14), 1840–42 (1993).

Levy, S. B., Burke, J. and Wallace, E. (eds), 'Antibiotic use and antibiotic resistance worldwide', *Review of Infectious Diseases* Vol. 9 Suppl. 3, 5231–316 (1987).

Mcleod, G., *A Veterinary Materia Medica*, Essex: Saffron Walden 1983.

Mare, I. J. and Coetze, J. N., 'The incidence of transmissible drug resistance factors among strains of *E. coli* in the Pretoria area', *South African Medical Journal* Vol. 40, 620–22 (1966).

Mare, I. J., 'Incidence of R-factors among Gram-negative bacteria in drug-free human and animal communities', *Nature* Vol. 220, 1046–7 (1968).

Monaghan, C. et al., 'Antibiotic resistance and R-factors in the faecal coliform flora of urban and rural dogs', *Antimicrobial Agents and Chemotherapy* (1981).

Ochiai, K., Totani, T. and Toshiki, Y., '*Shigella* strains resistant to three antibiotics. Epidemic caused by triply resistant *Shigella* strains in Nagoya', *Nihon Iji Shimpo* No. 1837, 25–37 (1959).

Ofek, I. et al., 'Anti *E. coli* adhesion activity of cranberry and blueberry juices', *New England Journal of Medicine* Vol. 324(22), 1599 (1991).

Schwalbe, R. S., Stapleton, J. T. and Gilligan, P. H., 'Emergence of vancomycin resistance in coagulase-negative *Staphylococci*', *New England Journal of Medicine* Vol. 316(15), 927–31 (1987).

Skurray, R. A., Rauch, D. A., Lyon, B. R. et al., 'Multi-resistant *Staphylococcus aureus*: genetics and evolution of epidemic Australian strains', *Journal of Antimicrobial Chemotherapy* Suppl. C, 19–39 (1988).

Swartz, W. et al., *Human health risks with the subtherapeutic use of penicillins or tetracyclines in animal feed*, Washington DC: National Academy Press 1989.

Welch, G. H., 'Antibiotic resistance: a new kind of epidemic', *Postgraduate Medicine* Vol. 6, 76 (1984).

Wolfe, S. M., 'Antibiotics', *Health Letter*, Washington DC: The Public Citizens Health Research Group 1989.

Chapter 3 The Use and Abuse of Antibiotics, pp. 29–39

Barnes, P. F. and Barrows, S. A., 'Tuberculosis in the 1990s', *Annals of Internal Medicine* Vol. 119(5), 400–410 (1993).

Cantekin, E. I. et al., 'Anti-microbial therapy for *Otitis media* with effusion', *Journal of the American Medical Association* Vol. 266(23), 3309–17 (1991).

Diamont, M. and Diamont, B., 'Abuse and timing of antibiotics in acute *Otitis media*', *Archives of Otolaryngology* Vol. 100, 226–32 (1974).

Hauser, W. E. and Remington, J. S., 'Effect of antibiotics on the immune system', *American Journal of Medicine* Vol. 72(5), 711–15 (1982).

Laurence, D. R and Bennett, P. N., *Clinical Pharmacology*, Edinburgh: Churchill Livingstone 1980.

Londymore-Lim, L., *Poisonous Prescriptions*, Australia: Prevention of Disease & Disability 1994.

Neu, H. C. and Henry, S. P., 'Testing the physician's knowledge of antibiotic use', *New England Journal of Medicine* Vol. 293, 1291 (1975).

Chapter 5 Childhood Infections, pp. 43–54

Bain, J., Murphy, E. and Ross, F., 'Acute *Otitis media*: clinical cause among children who received a short course of high-dose antibiotic', *British Medical Journal* Vol. 291, 1243–6 (1985).

Cantekin, E. I. et al., 'Anti-microbial therapy for *Otitis media* with effusion', *Journal of the American Medical Association* Vol. 266(23), 3309–17 (1991).

Freinberg, N. and Lyte, T., 'Adjunctive ascorbic acid administration and antibiotic therapy', *Journal of Dental Research* Vol. 36, 260–62 (1957).

Hull, D. and Johnston, D. I., *Essential Paediatrics*, Edinburgh: Churchill Livingstone 1981.

Kendig, E. L., *Disorders of the Respiratory Tract in Children*, Philadelphia: Saunders 1977.

Klein, J. O., 'Microbiology and Management of *Otitis media*', *Paediatrician* Vol. 8 Suppl. 1, 10–25 (1979).

Krugman, S., Ward, R. and Katz, S. L., *Infectious Diseases of Children*, St Louis: Mosby 1977.

Schmidt, M. A., *Childhood Ear Infections: What every parent and physician should know*, California: North Atlantic Books 1990.

Williams, H. E. and Phelan, P. D., *Respiratory Illness in Children*, Oxford: Blackwell Scientific 1975.

Chapter 6 Herbal Medicine, pp. 55–78

GENERAL

British Herbal Medicine Association Scientific Committee, *British Herbal Pharmacopoeia*, Vols. 1, 2 & 3, London: British Herbal Medicine Association 1983.

Mowrey, D. B., *The Scientific Validation of Herbal Medicine*, Connecticut: Keats Publishing 1986.

ECHINACEA

Coeugneit, E. and Kühnast, R., 'Recurrent *Candidiasis* adjuvant immuno-therapy with different formulations of Echinacea', *Therapiewoche* Vol. 36, 3352 (1986).

Freyer, H. U., 'Frequency of common infections in childhood and likelihood of prophylaxis', *Fortschritte der Therapie* Vol. 92, 165 (1974).

Hobbs, C., *The Echinacea Handbook*, California: Botanica Press 1989.

James, J., *AIDS Treatment News* Vol. 19 (1986).

Lloyd, J. U., *A Treatise on Echinacea*, Cincinnati: Lloyd Brothers 1917.

McLoughlin, G., 'Echinacea: A Literature Review', *Australian Journal of Medical Herbalism* Vol. 4, 104–11 (1992).

Wacker, A. and Hilbig, W., 'Virus inhibition by *Echinacea purpurea*', *Planta Medica* Vol. 33, 89 (1978).

WILD INDIGO (BAPTISIA)

Beuscher, N. and Kopanski, L., 'Stimulation of the immune response with substances derived from *Baptisia tinctoria*', *Planta Medica* Vol. 5, 381–4 (1985).

Beuscher, N., Beuscher, H. and Bodinet, C., 'Enhanced release of interleukin-I from mouse macrophages by glycoproteins and polysaccharides from *Baptisia tinctoria* and *Echinacea spp.*', *37th Annual Congress on Medicinal Plant Research*, Braunschweig 1989.

Culbreth, D., *A Manual of Materia Medica and Pharmacology*, Oregon: Ecletic Medical Publications 1983.

Moerman, D. E., *American Medical Ethno-botany*, New York: Garland Publishers 1977.

USNEA

Johnson, R. B. et al., 'The mode of action of the antibiotic, usnic acid', *Archives of Biochemistry and Biophysics* Vol. 28, 317–23 (1950).

Wagner, H. and Proksch, A., 'Immuno-stimulating drugs from fungi and higher plants' in *Progress in Medicinal and Economic Plant Research Vol. 1*, London: Academic Press 1983.

Weiss, R. F., *Herbal Medicine*, Beaconsfield: Beaconsfield Pub. 1988.

MYRRH AND OTHER MEDICINAL HERBS

Grieve, M., *A Modern Herbal*, New York: Dover 1971.

Wren, R. C. and Wren, R. W. (eds.), *Potter's New Cyclopaedia of Botanical Drugs and Preparations*, Holsworthy: Health Science Press 1975.

THUJA

Goullon, H., *Thuja occidentalis*, Leipzig: Gustav Engelverlag.

Halter, K., 'Innerliche Behandlung juveniler Warzen mit *Thuja occidentalis*', *Dermatologische Wochenschrift* Vol. 120, 353–5 (1949).

Khurana, S. M. P., 'Effect of homeopathic drugs on plant viruses', *Planta Medica* Vol. 20, 142–6 (1971).

Weiss, R. F., *Lehrbuch der Phytotherapie*, Stuttgart: Hippocrates Verlag 1980.

Chapter 7 Homeopathic Medicine, pp. 79–89

Campbell, A., *The Two Faces of Homeopathy*, London: Hale 1984.

Castro, D. and Nogueira, G., 'Use of the nosode meningococcinum as a preventive against meningitis', *Journal of the American Institute of Homeopathy* Vol. 68, 211–19 (1975).

Castro, M., *The Complete Homeopathy Handbook*, London: Macmillan 1990.

Coulter, H. L., *Homeopathic Science and Modern Medicine: The Physics of Healing with Microdoses*, California: North Atlantic Books 1987.

Gaucher, C., Jeulin, D. and Peycru, P., 'Homeopathic treatment of cholera in Peru: an initial clinical study', *British Homeopathic Journal* Vol. 81, 18–21 (1992).

Reckweg, H. H., *Materia Medica Homeopathica Anti-homotoxica*, Baden-Baden: Aurelia Verlag 1983.

Schmidt, M. A., Smith, L. H. and Sehnert, K. W., *Beyond Antibiotics*, California: North Atlantic Books 1993.

Tyler, M., *Homeopathic Drug Pictures*, London: Health Science Press 1970.

Vithoulkas, G., *Homeopathy: Medicine of the New Man*, Wellingborough: Thorsons 1985.

Vithoulkas, G., *The Science of Homeopathy*, Wellingborough: Thorsons 1986.

Chapter 8 Nutritional Medicine, pp. 90–107

GENERAL

Beukes, V., *Killer Foods of the Twentieth Century*, Johannesburg: Perskor 1974.

Bieler, H. M., *Food is Your Best Medicine*, London: Neville Spearman 1968.

Budd, M. L., *Low Blood Sugar (hypoglycaemia)—the 20th century epidemic?*, Wellingborough: Thorsons 1984.

Chavance, M. et al., 'Nutritional support improves antibody

response to influenza virus in the elderly', *British Medical Journal* Vol. 11(9), 1348–9 (1985).

Cheraskin, E., *Diet and Disease*, Connecticut: Keats Publishing 1968.

Kumar, A., Weatherly, M. and Beaman, D. C., 'Sweeteners, flavourings and dyes in antibiotic preparations', *Paediatrics* Vol. 87(3), 352–9 (1991).

Millstone, E. and Abraham, J., *Additives*, London: Penguin 1988.

Newberne, P. and Williams, G., 'Nutritional influences on the course of infections' in Dunlop, R. H. and Moon, H. W. (eds.), *Resistance to Infectious Disease*, Canada: Saskatoon Modern Press 1970.

Pfeiffer, C. C., *Total Nutrition*, London: Granada 1982.

Sanchez, A. et al., 'Role of sugar in human neutrophilic phagocytosis', *American Journal of Clinical Nutrition* Vol. 26, 180 (1973).

Sandler, B. P., *Diet Prevents Polio*, The Lee Foundation for Nutritional Research (1951).

Select Committee on Nutrition and Human Needs, *Dietary Goals for the United States*, Washington DC: U.S. Senate 1977.

Stitt, P. A., *Fighting the Food Giants*, Wisconsin: Natural Press 1980.

Vogel, H. C. A., *The Nature Doctor*, Edinburgh: Mainstream 1990.

Ward, N. I. et al., 'The influence of the chemical additive tartrazine on the zinc status of hyperactive children—a double-blind placebo-controlled study', *Journal of Nutritional Medicine* Vol. 1, 51–7 (1990).

Williams, R. J., *Nutrition Against Disease*, London: Pitman 1971.

Wilson, F. A., *Food Fit for Humans*, London: Daniel 1975.

LIVE YOGHURT

Alm, I., Leiyenmark, C. E., Persson, A. K. and Midvedt, T., 'The Regulatory and Protective Role of the Normal Microflora', *Wenner-Gren International Symposium Series* (1988).

Barefoot, S. and Klaenhammer, T. R., 'Detection and activity of Lactacin B, a bacteriocin produced by *Lactobacillus acidophilus*', *Applied and Environmental Microbiology* Vol. 45, 1808 (1983).

Bullen, C. L., Tearle, P. V. and Willis, A. T., 'Bifidobacteria in the intestinal tract of infants: an *in vivo* study', *Journal of Medical Microbiology* Vol. 9, 325 (1975).

Byssen, H., 'Role of the gut micro-flora in metabolism of lipids and sterols', *Proceedings of the Nutrition Society* Vol. 32, 59 (1973).

Colombel, J. F., Cartol, A., Newt, C. and Romond, C., 'Yoghurt with *Bifidobacterium longum* reduces erythromycin-induced gastro-intestinal effects', *The Lancet* Vol. 2, 43 (1987).

Goldin, B. R. and Gorbach, S. L., 'Alterations of the intestinal flora by diet, oral antibiotics and *Lactobacillus*', *Journal of the National Cancer Institute* Vol. 73, 689 (1984).

Gordon, D., Macrea, J. and Wheater, D. M., 'A *Lactobacillus* preparation for use with antibiotics', *The Lancet* Vol. 272, 889 (1957).

Hamdan, I. T. et al. 'Acidolin: an antibiotic produced by *Lactobacillus acidophilus*', *Journal of Antibiotics* Vol. 27, 631 (1974).

Kim, H. S. and Gilliland, S. E., '*Lactobacillus acidophilus* as a dietary adjunct for milk to aid lactose digestion in humans', *Journal of Dairy Science* Vol. 66, 959 (1983).

Lipid Research Clinics Program, 'The lipid research clinics coronary primary prevention trials results: Reduction in the incidence of coronary heart disease', *Journal of the American Medical Association* Vol. 251, 351 (1984).

Mann, G. V., 'A factor in yoghurt which lowers cholesteremia in man', *Atherosclerosis* Vol. 26(3), 335–40 (1977).

Mann, G. V. and Spoerry, A., 'Studies of a surfactant and cholesteremia in the Masai', *American Journal of Clinical Nutrition* Vol. 27, 464 (1974).

Shahani, K. M. and Ayebo, A., 'Role of dietary *lactobacilli* in the gastro-intestinal microecology', *American Journal of Clinical Nutrition* Vol. 33, 2448 (1980).

Chapter 9 Nutritional Supplements, pp. 108–19

VITAMIN C (PERIODICALS)

Anderson, R. et al., 'The effects of increasing weekly doses of ascorbate on certain cellular and hormonal immune functions in normal volunteers', *American Journal of Clinical Nutrition* Vol. 33, 71 (1980).

Beisel, W., Edelman, R. et al., 'Single nutrient effects of immunologic function', *Journal of the American Medical Association* Vol. 245, 53–8 (1981).

Bright-See, E., 'Vitamin C and cancer prevention', *Seminars in Oncology* Vol. 10(3), 294–8 (1983).

Cameron, E. and Pauling, L., 'Supplemental ascorbate in the supportive treatment of cancer: prolongation of survival times in terminal human cancer', *Proceedings of the National Academy of Sciences* Vol. 73, 3685 (1976).

Dahl, H. and Degre, M., 'The effect of ascorbic acid on the production of human interferon and the anti-viral activity *in vitro*', *Acta Pathologica, Microbiologica et Immunologica Scandinavia B* Vol. 84, 280 (1976).

Dieter, M., 'Further studies on the relationship between vitamin C and thymic hormonal factor', *Proceedings of the Society for Experimental Biology and Medicine* Vol. 136, 316–22 (1971).

Fraser, R. C. et al., 'The effect of variations in vitamin C intake on the cellular response of guinea pigs', *American Journal of Clinical Nutrition* Vol. 33, 839 (1980).

Frei, B., England. L. and Ames, B. N., 'Ascorbate as an outstanding antioxidant in human blood plasma', *Proceedings of the National Academy of Sciences* Vol. 86, 6377 (1989).

Hoffer, A., 'Ascorbic acid and kidney stones', *Canadian Medical Association Journal* Vol. 132, 320 (1985).

Karlowski, T. R. et al., 'Ascorbic acid for the common cold: A prophylactic and therapeutic trial', *Journal of the American Medical Association* Vol. 231, 1038 (1975).

Kaul, T. N., Middleton, E. and Orga, P., 'Antiviral effect of flavinoids on human viruses', *Journal of Medical Virology* Vol. 15, 71–9 (1985).

Klein, M. A., 'The National Cancer Institute and ascorbic acid', *Townsend Letter for Doctors* (1991).

Klenner, F. R., 'Virus pneumonia and its treatment with vitamin C', *Journal of Southern Medicine and Surgery* Vol. 2 (1948).

Klenner, F. R., 'Massive doses of vitamin C and the virus diseases', *Journal of Southern Medicine and Surgery* Vol. 113(4) (1951).

Klenner, F. R., 'The use of vitamin C as an antibiotic', *Journal of Applied Nutrition* Vol. 6 (1953).

Leibovitz, B. and Siegel, B. V., 'Ascorbic acid, neutrophil function and the immune system', *International Journal of Vitamin and Nutrition Research* Vol. 48, 159 (1978).

Pauling, L., 'Evolution and the need for ascorbic acid', *Proceedings of the National Academy of Sciences* Vol. 67, 1643 (1970).

Pauling, L., 'The significance of the evidence about ascorbic acid and the common cold', *Proceedings of the National Academy of Sciences* Vol. 68, 2678–81 (1971).

Rivers, J. M., 'Safety of high level vitamin C ingestion', Applied Nutrition 3rd Conference on Vitamin C, *Annals of the New York Academy of Science* Vol. 498, 445–54 (1987).

Romney, S. L. et al., 'Plasma vitamin C and uterine cervical dysplasia', *American Journal of Obstetrics and Gynecology* Vol. 151, 976–80 (1985).

Scott, J., 'On the biochemical similarities of ascorbic acid and interferon', *Journal of Theoretical Biology* Vol. 98, 235–8 (1982).

Shilotri, P. G. and Bhat, K. S., 'Effect of megadoses of vitamin C on bactericidal activity of leukocytes', *American Journal of Clinical Nutrition* Vol. 30, 1077 (1977).

Siegel, B. V. and Morton, J. I., 'Vitamin C and immunity: Influence of ascorbate on PGE2 synthesis and implications for natural killer cell activity', *International Journal of Vitamin and Nutrition Research* Vol. 54, 339 (1984).

Siegel, B. V., 'Enhanced interferon response to murine leukaemia virus by ascorbic acid', *Infection and Immunity* Vol. 10, 409 (1974).

VITAMIN C (BOOKS)

Cheraskin, E., Ringsdorf, W. M. and Sisley, E. L., *The Vitamin C Connection*, Wellingborough: Thorsons 1983.

Hornig, D., *Vitamins and Minerals in Pregnancy and Lactation: Nestlé Nutrition Workshop Series*, No. 16, 433–4, New York: Raven Press 1988.

Kalokerinos, A., *Every Second Child*, Connecticut: Keats Publishing 1981.

Pauling, L., *How to live longer and feel better*, New York: W. H. Freeman 1986.

Pauling, L., *Vitamin C and the Common Cold*, San Francisco: W. H. Freeman 1970.

Stone, I., *The Healing Factor: Vitamin C against Disease*, New York: Gromet & Dunlop 1972.

ZINC

Al-Nakib, M., Higgins, P. G., Barrow, I. et al., 'Prophylaxis and treatment of rhinovirus colds with zinc gluconate lozenges', *Journal of Antimicrobial Chemotherapy* Vol. 20, 893–901 (1987).

Bogden, J. D., Oleske, J. M., Munves, E. M. et al., 'Zinc and immunocompetence in the elderly: baseline data on zinc and immunity in unsupplemental subjects', *American Journal of Clinical Nutrition* Vol. 46, 101–9 (1987).

Brody, I., 'Topical treatment of recurrent *herpes simplex* and post-herpetic erythema multiforme with low concentrations of zinc sulphate solution', *British Journal of Dermatology* Vol. 104, 191–4 (1981).

Bulkena, E. G., 'Zinc compounds, a new treatment in peptic ulcer', *Drugs under Experimental and Clinical Research* Vol. 15(2), 83–9 (1989).

Chandra, R. K., 'Excessive intake of zinc impairs immune responses', *Journal of the American Medical Association* Vol. 252, 1443–6 (1984).

Duchateau, J. et al., 'Beneficial effects of oral zinc supplementation on the immune response of old people', *American Journal of Medicine* Vol. 70, 1001–4 (1981).

Eby, G. A., Davis, D. A. and Halcomb, W. W., 'Reduction in duration of common colds by zinc gluconate lozenges in a double-blind study', *Antimicrobial Agents and Chemotherapy* Vol. 25, 20 (1984).

Fabris, N. et al., 'AIDS, zinc deficiency and thymic hormone failure', *Journal of the American Medical Association* Vol. 259, 839–40 (1988).

Hansen, M. A., Fernandes, G. and Good, R. A., 'Nutrition and Immunity: The influence of diet on auto-immunity and the role of zinc in the immune response', *Annual Review of Nutrition* Vol. 2, 151–77 (1982).

Katz, E. and Margolith, E., 'Inhibition of vaccinia virus maturation by zinc chloride', *Antimicrobial Agents and Chemotherapy* Vol. 19, 213–7 (1981).

Prasar, A., 'Clinical biochemical and nutritional spectrum of zinc deficiency in human subjects: an update', *Nutrition Review* Vol. 41, 197–208 (1983).

Chapter 10 The Role of Stress, pp. 120–34

Angier, N., 'Chronic anger is a major health risk: studies find', *New York Times* (13 December 1990) (from papers presented at the 1990 conference of the American Heart Association).

Benson, H., *The Relaxation Response*, New York: Morrow 1975.

Bombardelli, E., Cirstoni, A. and Liehi, A., 'The effect of acute and chronic ginseng saponins treatment on adrenal function', *Proceedings of the 3rd International Ginseng Symposium* (1980).

Boyce, T. W. et al., 'Influence of life events and family routines on childhood respiratory tract illness', *Paediatrics* Vol. 60(4), 609–15 (1977).

Cohen, S., Tyrrell, D. and Smith, A., 'Psychological stress and susceptibility to the common cold', *New England Journal of Medicine* Vol. 325, 606–12 (1991).

D'Angelo, L., Grimaldi, R., Carravaggi, M. et al., 'A double-blind placebo controlled clinical study on the effect of a standardised ginseng extract on psychomotor performance in healthy volunteers', *Journal of Ethnopharmacology* Vol. 16, 15–22 (1986).

Fulder, S. J., 'Ginseng and the hypothalamic-pituitary control of stress', *American Journal of Chinese Medicine* Vol. 9, 112–18 (1981).

Hoffman, D., *The New Holistic Herbal*, London: Element 1990.

Holmes, T. H. and Rahe, R. H., 'The Social Readjustment Scale', *Journal of Psychosomatic Research* Vol. 11, 213–18 (1967). [Reproduced with permission].

Moldofsky, H. et al., 'The relationship of interleukin-I and immune functions to sleep in humans', *Psychosomatic Medicine* Vol. 48, 309–15 (1986).

Pizzorno, J. E. and Murray, M. T., *A Textbook of Natural Medicine*, California: Prima 1988.

Seyle, H., *Stress in Health and Disease*, London: Butterworths 1976.

Simonton, O. C., Matthews-Simonton, S. and Creighton, J. L., *Getting Well Again*, London: Bantam 1980.

Sobel, D. and Ornstein, R., *Healthy Pleasures*, Massachusetts: Addison-Wesley 1989.

Index

152